APPLIED
PHLEBOTOMY

APPLIED
PHLEBOTOMY

DENNIS J. ERNST

 LIPPINCOTT WILLIAMS & WILKINS
A **Wolters Kluwer** Company

Philadelphia • Baltimore • New York • London
Buenos Aires • Hong Kong • Sydney • Tokyo

Acquisitions Editor: Pamela Lappies
Managing Editor: Kevin C. Dietz
Marketing Manager: Mary Martin
Associate Production Manager: Kevin Johnson
Designer: Teresa Mallon
Compositor: Maryland Composition, Inc.
Printer: RR Donnelley-Crawfordsville

The publisher is not responsible (as a matter of product liability, negligence, or otherwise) for any injury resulting from any material contained herein. This publication contains information relating to general principles of medical care that should not be construed as specific instructions for individual patients. Manufacturers' product information and package inserts should be reviewed for current information, including contraindications, dosages, and precautions.

Printed in the United States of America

Library of Congress Cataloging-in-Publication Data

Ernst, Dennis J., MT(ASCP)
    Applied phlebotomy / Dennis J. Ernst.
        p. ; cm.
    Includes bibliographical references and index.
    ISBN 0-7817-5055-5
    1. Phlebotomy.   I. Title. [DNLM: 1. Phlebotomy—adverse effects.   2. Phlebotomy—instrumentation.   3. Phlebotomy—methods.   4. Medical Errors—prevention & control.
5. Risk Assessment.   6. Specimen Handling—methods.]
    RB45.15.E758 2005
    616.07′561—dc22

                                                                                    2005001797

The publishers have made every effort to trace the copyright holders for borrowed material. If they have inadvertently overlooked any, they will be pleased to make the necessary arrangements at the first opportunity.

To purchase additional copies of this book, call our customer service department at (800) 638-3030 or fax orders to (301) 824-7390. International customers should call (301) 714-2324.

Visit Lippincott Williams & Wilkins on the Internet: http://www.LWW.com. Lippincott Williams & Wilkins customer service representatives are available from 8:30 am to 6:00 pm, EST.

06 07
1 2 3 4 5 6 7 8 9 10

To my loving wife, Catherine,
for her unfailing support and encouragement.

REVIEWERS

Christopher J. Rasmussen, MS
Research Coordinator/Part-time Lecturer
Exercise & Sport Nutrition Laboratory
Baylor University
Waco, Texas

Laine K. Stewart, CLS (NCA), MT (ASCP)
Clinical Laboratory Science Instructor
University of North Carolina at Chapel Hill
Chapel Hill, North Carolina

Janet L. Vincent, MS, SBB (ASCP)
Education Coordinator
University of Texas Medical Branch
Department of Pathology
Galveston, Texas

Whitney Williams, PhD, MT (ASCP)
Program Director
Clinical Laboratory Sciences Program
Arkansas State University
Jonesboro, Arkansas

PREFACE

It has been said that phlebotomy is the most underestimated procedure in healthcare. To the casual observer, those with experience make the procedure look deceptively simple. This misconception has, in large part, contributed to the trend in healthcare to assign blood collection responsibilities to healthcare professionals outside of the clinical laboratory. Today, the allied healthcare professionals who are called upon to perform blood collection procedures include not only laboratory-based phlebotomists and technical personnel, but nurses, nursing assistants, respiratory care technicians, emergency room technicians, medical assistants, physician's assistants, paramedics, emergency medical technicians, and patient care technicians.

The risk in underestimating phlebotomy is significant and potentially devastating to patients. Inadequate training can cause collectors to corrupt specimens during the collection process, leading to results that do not reflect the patient's true physiology. Inaccurate results can cause physicians to overmedicate, undermedicate, misdiagnose, or otherwise mismanage their patients, resulting in serious complications, including death. Additionally, improperly trained specimen collection personnel can inflict injuries to patients during the procedure. Therefore, it is important to demonstrate just how complex a "simple" venipuncture can be.

It is the goal of *Applied Phlebotomy* to dispel the myth that anyone can draw blood specimens properly with just a few hours of basic training. In this text evidence to the contrary is presented in the form of case studies of actual patients who have been permanently injured, disfigured, or disabled at the hands of those who take a cavalier approach to phlebotomy or were trained by those who failed to take phlebotomy seriously. It is a primary objective of this text to immunize the reader against inflicting a potentially disabling injury and the legal proceedings that often follow by bringing to light the common mistakes healthcare professionals make during specimen collection procedures that lead to injury and litigation.

This text is intended to provide those who train and educate all healthcare professionals with a resource that can serve as the backbone of their phlebotomy training program in: (1) healthcare facilities, including hospitals, clinics, surgery centers, reference laboratories, etc; and (2) allied healthcare programs at colleges, universities, and vocational schools.

In addition, this book strives to be a source of current and accurate information for today's healthcare worker who is currently performing blood collection procedures in any capacity.

Every passage, illustration, chart, table, and reference has been prepared to teach blood collection procedures and practices that safeguard healthcare workers from accidental exposures, protect patients from injury, and yield specimens that are free of collection and processing errors that alter results. To that end, this text has been painstakingly researched to reflect the current standards of the Clinical and Laboratory Standards Institute (formerly

NCCLS) on specimen collection, the current OSHA guidelines on preventing employee injury, and the current recommendations on infection control and risk management.

Four special features that will enhance your understanding include:

- In the Lab
- It Could Happen to You
- According to the Standards
- Tips from the Trenches

The "In the Lab" sections explain why certain procedures and theories are important to specimen collection by describing how specimens are processed in the clinical laboratory, and how they can significantly impact patient care if improperly collected. The "It Could Happen to You" feature details actual case studies of phlebotomy-related injuries to illustrate key concepts and learning objectives. "Tips from the Trenches" apply concepts to real-life situations. Finally, the "According to the Standards" feature calls attention to important passages from the Clinical and Laboratory Standards Institute (formerly NCCLS) documents that should be incorporated into everyone's technique and reflected in every blood collection procedure manual.

Additional features of this text include:

- End-of-chapter quizzes for evaluating comprehension and preparing for certification exams
- The latest Centers for Disease Control recommendations for exposure evaluation and treatment
- Comprehensive appendices listing educational resources, certification organizations, and online resources

Because this text is for the allied healthcare practitioner and advanced student, a working knowledge of basic body systems, medical terminology, phlebotomy theory and principles, clinical diagnosis by laboratory methods, anatomy, physiology, and healthcare delivery is assumed. A working knowledge of healthcare and the clinical laboratory's contribution to patient care are anticipated. Many excellent texts already exist for those without a background in healthcare. Instead, this book is designed to provide practicing healthcare professionals and advanced allied healthcare educators with a tool for cross-training laboratory professionals and to provide laboratory phlebotomists, managers, and educators with the most current and authoritative text on the subject of phlebotomy.

Acknowledgments

I would like to thank Warren Lynch and Associates for paying such great attention to detail while photographing the images for this text. Thanks also to the many companies who have provided images, including Greiner Bio-One, Medi-Flex, and Life-Tech. Special thanks to Ruth Carrico for sharing her expertise in infection control and exposure management.

TABLE OF CONTENTS

Phlebotomy: Not Just a Procedure Anymore

1

INTRODUCTION

Before it was even called phlebotomy, practitioners of the healing arts accessed veins for the purpose of bloodletting, which was thought to be therapeutic. The draining of blood to rid the body of disease and restore balance has ancient origins. Historians tell us that George Washington died after being bled excessively during a 2-day period in an attempt to cure a cold. Today, phlebotomy (from the Greek words *phlebos* [veins] and *tome* [to cut]) serves a different purpose. Although therapeutic phlebotomy is still performed in patients with polycythmia rubra vera, hemochromocytosis, and other conditions to reduce an excessively high concentration of circulating red blood cells, phlebotomy is performed primarily to obtain specimens for clinical testing to assist physicians in the management of their patients' health.

This chapter will introduce the reader to the role of phlebotomy in healthcare and assess the current status of phlebotomy in today's healthcare setting. For managers, it will identify strategies to manage the risks phlebotomy brings to a facility and to the individuals who perform blood collection procedures. To that end, a discussion on minimum training requirements is provided to assist in administering an effective training program. Other management sections will assist managers in drafting procedures that infuse safety, inspire professionalism, and nurture a culture of customer service. For those who draw specimens for clinical testing, projecting a positive image is paramount to gaining patient confidence and satisfaction. Because a positive patient experience is as essential to a successful procedure as technique, customer service skills and professional development are discussed at length.

After completing this chapter, the reader should be able to:

- Discuss the role of phlebotomy in healthcare
- Describe the evolution of phlebotomy in healthcare
- Develop a comprehensive in-house phlebotomy training program
- Draft phlebotomy procedures that infuse safety
- Inspire professionalism among those with blood collection responsibilities

- Develop a culture of customer service among phlebotomists
- Appreciate the importance of personal appearance to the patient's perception of the testing facility
- List the essential elements of telephone etiquette
- Associate phlebotomy certification with professionalism
- Project a professional image to patients and co-workers

EVOLUTION OF PHLEBOTOMY IN HEALTHCARE

Staffing Strategies

Before the 1970s, laboratorians with certification as Medical Technologists and their assistants were responsible for drawing blood specimens from patients for clinical testing. As the cost to employ certified laboratory personnel increased, so did the pressure from administrators and chief financial officers to utilize them more cost-effectively. The mantra: keep higher-paid testing personnel in the testing environment, conducting the technical aspects of laboratory medicine that they were trained to do, and create lower-paying positions to draw and prepare the specimens to be tested. These specimen collection personnel, known as phlebotomists, became essential members of the clinical laboratory staff.

Through the 1970s and 1980s, phlebotomists honed their skills while the technical personnel sharpened their focus on analysis. With the costs of healthcare continuing to spiral out of control, the 1990s ushered in a new management mantra: convert one-skill phlebotomists to multiskilled "patient care assistants." Based on the premise that healthcare personnel are more efficient when they are capable of performing multiple tasks, phlebotomists who had mastered the art of specimen collection became cross-trained to take vital signs, ambulate patients, bathe patients, and perform other patient care functions. With the additional responsibilities came a relocation of the phlebotomist from one department to another. The new "patient care associate" (PCA) was relocated from the laboratory to the nursing floors and assigned to the nursing staff. Dissatisfied with the uprooting, many skilled phlebotomists left the healthcare profession completely. Others adapted.

To the patient, however, the quality of venipunctures performed on them deteriorated substantially. Patients experienced multiple, painful, repeat punctures and excessively traumatized venipuncture sites. Satisfaction surveys plummeted. Laboratories noted deterioration in specimen quality and a dramatic increase in unacceptable specimens. Efficiencies gained in the redeployment of phlebotomists to the nursing staff were lost by delays in testing and the cost of recollecting specimens that arrived underfilled, hemolyzed, mislabeled, incorrectly collected, or otherwise unacceptable for testing (1,2).

Because the attempt to streamline the work force appeared to be misguided on many accounts, many administrators became convinced that the patient, and therefore the facility, was best served by bringing blood collection practices back within the control of the laboratory and reinstituting laboratory-based phlebotomy positions. Others remained firmly entrenched in the decentralized phlebotomy experiment. Some facilities found success in hybrid phlebotomy staffing strategies. One institution experienced such a decline in the quality of their specimen collection services that they instituted a "clinical technician" position (3). The clinical technician was laboratory-based and responsible for specimen collection, intravenous (IV) insertion, Holter monitor application, and ECGs. Under the clinical technician model, the percentage of early morning specimens received in the laboratory by 7 a.m. increased from 50% to 90%, and the specimen rejection rate dropped to less than 0.5%. Administrators realized a cost savings of $400,000.

Phlebotomy in a Multiskilled Work Force

Today, blood specimens are still drawn by a wide variety of healthcare professionals: nurses, physicians, nursing assistants, respiratory therapists, emergency department technicians, patient-care associates, emergency medical technicians, paramedics, medical assistants, and phlebotomists. Because phlebotomy is only one of many responsibilities for many healthcare professionals, the level of field expertise varies substantially. In a multiskilled work force, phlebotomy expertise is directly proportional to the frequency of performance and length of training. The challenge to administrators of a multiskilled work force is to provide adequate training to those for whom blood collection is one of many skills (Fig. 1.1).

Historically, the degree to which phlebotomy impacts patient care and the extent of training necessary to perform the procedure properly have been underestimated. Contributing to the misconception is that to the casual observer a venipuncture appears to be an outwardly simple procedure. Contributing to the illusion of simplicity is the fact that the effect improper technique has on the patient, through an inaccurate result, is often delayed or never directly attributed to collection errors. Most investigations of questionable results focus on the testing phase first and the preanalytical phase second, making collection technique twice removed from negative patient outcomes. For example, it is well known that when a tourniquet is applied

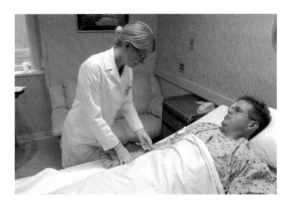

FIGURE 1.1 Today, blood specimens are drawn by a vide variety of healthcare professions

longer than 1 minute, changes begin to occur in the blood pooling below the constriction including an increase in the measurable potassium level. When those who draw blood specimens are subjected to an abbreviated training program, this fundamental may not be taught. As a result, drawing blood from a presurgery patient may produce a potassium level that is erroneously elevated. If the patient's actual potassium level is too low for surgery, but elevated to a normal level by of a prolonged tourniquet application, the patient may develop seizures and other complications, including death, while in surgery. Tracing the death back to the tourniquet error would be virtually impossible.

If phlebotomy was indeed a simple procedure, this and many other similar scenarios caused by poorly performed venipunctures would not be possible. Nor would it be possible for healthcare personnel to inflict the multitude of nerve injuries that occur during needle insertion every year (see Chapter 7). Because phlebotomy is easily underestimated and the impact of the collection technique on the result is twice removed, healthcare personnel and administrators without a laboratory background find it easy to consider specimen collection benign.

A common misperception among the nursing profession is that drawing blood is similar to inserting an IV. In fact, the two procedures are vastly different. Using the same technique for drawing a blood specimen as one uses to start an IV not only risks injury to the patient, but ignores the multitude of effects the procedure has on the specimen and ultimately the test results. As a result of this and other misperceptions, more and more healthcare personnel are being given blood collection responsibilities without adequate training (Fig. 1.2). The challenge for administrators managing a multiskilled work force is to provide the training commensurate with the potential impact the procedure has on patient care and those assigned blood collection responsibilities. It begins with understanding that impact. See Table 1.1 for a partial list of negative outcomes that can occur when specimens are obtained by personnel with inadequate training.

 Tips from the Trenches: *Administrators managing a multiskilled work force should provide training commensurate with the potential impact the procedure has on patient care and those assigned blood collection responsibilities.*

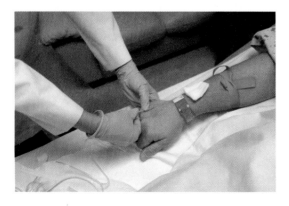

FIGURE 1.2 A common misperception among the nursing profession is that drawing blood is similar to inserting an IV.

TABLE 1.1 ■ Risks of Phlebotomy

The following risks to patient and collector underscore the importance of a comprehensive training program for all healthcare personnel who are given blood collection responsibilities. Each of these negative outcomes exposes the employer to the risk of litigation.

Preanalytical Errors	Negative Patient Outcome
Failure to properly identify the patient or label the specimen	Transfusion- or medication-related death. Patient mismanagement
Underfilling collection tube	Coag tube: Stroke/hemorrhage due to unnecessary modification of blood thinner dosage
	EDTA tube: Patient mismanagement from falsely decreased results
Additive carry-over due to incorrect order of draw	Cardiac arrhythmia
	Seizure and death due to falsely elevated potassium level
Specimen was not protected from light	Falsely lower result prevents physician intervention. Newborn suffers irreversible brain damage
Underfilling blood culture bottles	Death from septicemia due to false-negative result
Failure to properly cleanse venipuncture site	False-positive blood culture leads to unnecessary administration of antibiotic/extended length of hospitalization
Prolonged tourniquet application	Seizure and death due to falsely elevated potassium level
	Cardiac arrhythmia
	Undetected anemia
Failure to inquire about patient allergies to latex	Sensitization/Anaphylactic shock
Failure to label the specimen at the patient's side	Transfusion- or medication-related death. Patient mismanagement
Pouring contents of one tube into another	Stroke/hemorrhage due to unnecessary modification of blood thinner dosage. Patient mismanagement from altered results
Delay in transporting/testing coagulation specimens	Stroke/hemorrhage due to modification of blood thinner dosage based on inaccurate aPTT result
Delay in separating serum from cells	Seizure and death due to falsely elevated potassium level.
	Cardiac arrhythmia
	Patient mismanagement
Patient allowed to pump fist	Cardiac arrhythmia
	Seizure and death due to falsely elevated potassium level
	Patient mismanagement
Specimen drawn above IV	Patient death/mismanagement
Inadequate discard volume drawn when collecting blood through vascular access device	Stroke/hemorrhage due to modification of blood thinner dosage based on inaccurate coagulation results. Patient mismanagement from altered results
Errors That Injure Patients	**Negative Patient Outcome**
Arterial nick and/or inadequate pressure applied to venipuncture site	Hemorrhage that leads to nerve injury, compartment syndrome or limb amputation
Lack of knowledge of the anatomy of the antecubital area	Permanent, disabling nerve injuries
Bandage applied to heelstick	Newborn choking death
Failure to anticipate syncope	Fractures, contusions, concussions, paralysis

(continues)

TABLE 1.1 ■ Risks of Phlebotomy (continued)

Errors That Injure Patients	Negative Patient Outcome
Failure to inquire about patient allergies to latex	Sensitization/anaphylactic shock
Drawing from the side of a mastectomy	Lymphedema
Excessive needle manipulation	Permanent, disabling nerve injuries/arterial laceration
Failure to survey both arms for medial vein	Impaling median nerve while attempting to access basilic vein when safer vein was available/permanent nerve injury
Failure to use a tourniquet	Permanent nerve injury while attempting to access basilic vein when safer vein was available, but not made evident
Excessive angle of needle insertion	Needle penetrates through vein, into nerve or artery
	Permanent, disabling nerve injuries/arterial puncture
Failure to remove needle upon shooting pain sensation	Permanent, disabling nerve injuries
Errors That Cause Employee Injury	**Negative Employee Outcome**
Accidental needlestick	Acquiring HIV, hepatitis, or any of 20 diseases known to be transmitted by blood exposure
Exposure to breaks in skin from drawing or processing blood without gloves,	Acquiring HIV, hepatitis, or any of 20 diseases known to be transmitted by blood exposure
Repeated use of latex gloves/tourniquets	Sensitization/anaphylactic shock
Improper ergonomics when positioning patient	Back injuries

Providing adequate training for all healthcare professions assigned blood collection responsibilities helps ensure accurate results and minimizes the negative outcomes that can easily occur when physicians diagnose and manage their patients based on results adulterated during the collection process. In 2002, the state of California formally recognized the importance of a comprehensive phlebotomy training program when it regulated that all phlebotomists become certified and that those without experience undergo 80 hours of training followed by 50 supervised venipunctures. Other states are considering similar legislation.

When venipunctures are performed by a properly trained staff, patients are less likely to suffer direct injuries or treatments based on inaccurate results. For laboratories to report consistently accurate results it is critical that managers and administrators:

- Establish and maintain high standards for specimen collection personnel
- Fully understand the impact that an inadequately trained staff can have on patient care

Phlebotomy as a Nursing Procedure: An Historical Perspective

In the history of hospital-based healthcare, specimen collection began as a laboratory function. It made sense for those testing the blood to have control over all aspects of the specimen, including its collection. Then, in the 1970s, laboratories sensed a need to streamline their work flow and created blood collection specialists—phlebotomists—to collect and process specimens. Creating this position allowed the higher paid laboratory technologists to concentrate on the highly technical testing phase of clinical laboratory work. Because blood collection and its processing were their only responsibilities, phlebotomists perfected the technique and became highly skilled members of the healthcare team.

However, as America's monstrously wasteful healthcare delivery machine lumbered through the 1980s and into the 1990s, healthcare providers were forced to take a hard look at the economics of their staffing patterns. To those who were responsible for keeping facilities solvent, it became increasingly obvious that employing individuals who have only one skill was an inefficient use of human resources. While it was true that phlebotomists allowed the higher paid laboratorians to concentrate on specimen analysis, those who weren't performing other laboratory functions in between venipunctures accumulated hours and hours of downtime, the elimination of which became the mantra of healthcare administrators, chief financial officers, and human resources directors industry-wide. Adding even more pressure to modify the role of the phlebotomist, patient satisfaction surveys began to show that the more employees that patients encountered during their stay, the less satisfied they were with their care. This urged administrators to move phlebotomists to the bedside as caregivers capable of performing other direct patient care functions. Adding more appeal was the opportunity it presented to reduce their work force (a perpetual objective) by combining positions. This restructuring concept threatened the demise of the one-skill, laboratory-based phlebotomist.

Gradually, the terms "cross-trained" and "multiskilled" echoed from the boardrooms and hallways to define those who could be trained to perform a multitude of formerly foreign functions. Despite evidence of a negative impact on the quality of care, the trend continues not only to make phlebotomy the responsibility of the newly designated "patient care associates" (or some similar variation), but to add blood collection procedures to the list of duties of the already overburdened nurse.

In long-term care facilities the transition of phlebotomy to a nursing-based function has other origins. Reference laboratories are under increasing pressure to eliminate their phlebotomy services to their clients. The practice of providing free phlebotomy services in exchange for a facility's agreement to use their labs for reference work is now illegal in many cases. The Prospective Payment System enacted by Medicare makes it difficult for reference labs to provide this service even for a fee. Therefore, facilities for the aged are being forced to make other arrangements to have their residents' specimens collected. For most, the logical solution is to train their employees to collect the specimens themselves. Unfortunately, many facilities don't have the resources to train their staff to perform phlebotomy properly.

The industry continues to debate the wisdom of these transitions in theory and in practice.

(Reprinted from Ernst DJ, Ernst C. *Phlebotomy for Nurses and Nursing Personnel*. Ramsey, IN: HealthStar Press, 2001, with permission.)

PHLEBOTOMY'S ROLE IN HEALTHCARE

As in most manufacturing processes, the quality of the end product is dependent upon the quality of the materials that go into its creation and the skill of those who create it. In healthcare, the product is health. A key component of health is the information the physician receives on the patient's well-being. Seventy percent of the objective information the physician receives on the patient's status comes from the results of tests performed by the clinical laboratory on blood and other body fluids (4). A test result, therefore, is a product of the laboratory that physicians rely on heavily to establish and maintain the health of their patients.

 Tips from the Trenches: *Specimen collection personnel who understand that 70% of the objective information the physician receives on the patient's status comes from results obtained from specimens collected for laboratory testing are more likely to perform specimen collection procedures according to the standards.*

With so much dependent on the accuracy of the test result, laboratory processes have been extensively studied and perfected to eliminate sources of error. As a laboratory product, the quality of the test result is partially dependent on precise laboratory instrumentation and the skill of testing personnel. Sophisticated instrumentation and highly sensitive test methodologies are now available that have eliminated many of the sources of error that could alter results. Studies show that of all the errors that can affect the quality of a test result, only 13% occur during the testing (analytical) phase (5,6). However, even the most sophisticated testing instrumentation and most highly skilled testing personnel cannot extract an accurate result from a specimen that has not been collected and/or processed properly. Because specimen collection and processing can never be fully automated, up to 56% of the errors that can alter test results occur during this "preanalytical" phase. (See Chapter 6, "Specimen Handling and Storage.") As a result, preanalytical errors cost the average 400-bed hospital $200,000 per year in recollections and medication errors (7). When specimen collection and processing errors contribute to a low-quality test result, the ultimate product the healthcare industry delivers, patient health, can be tragically flawed. Table 1.1 illustrates some of the risks associated with specimen collection and processing that adversely affect the health of the patient and the collector.

 Tips from the Trenches: *Up to 56% of the errors that can alter test results occur during the specimen collection and processing phase of clinical testing.*

Because phlebotomy will always be a manual procedure, it is critical to properly educate and supervise those with blood collection responsibilities to prevent the high number of possible errors from becoming actual errors that lead to negative patient outcomes. For the same reason, those properly trained to draw blood specimens must diligently adhere to the standards and their facility's policies to ensure that testing personnel can extract an accurate result from the specimen (Fig. 1.3).

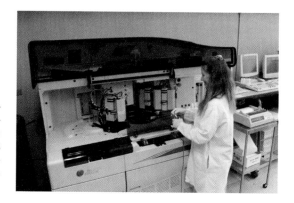

FIGURE 1.3 No degree of sophisticated instrumentation or expertise of testing personnel can obtain a result that reflects the patient's actual health status from a specimen altered by improper collection and/or processing

No degree of sophisticated instrumentation or expertise of testing personnel can obtain a result that reflects the patient's actual health status from a specimen altered by improper collection and/or processing. Some preanalytical errors can be detected by testing personnel, but most cannot. These undetected errors can contribute to erroneous results and cause physicians to misdiagnose, overmedicate, undermedicate, and mismanage their patients. Therefore, those who draw specimens have significant influence on 70% of the objective information physicians receive on patient health status. The importance of specimen collection cannot be overstated.

 Tips from the Trenches: No degree of sophisticated instrumentation or expertise of testing personnel can obtain a result that reflects the patient's actual health status from a specimen altered by improper collection and/or processing.

IDENTIFYING AND MANAGING THE RISKS

Treating patients according to results that are inaccurate due to poor specimen collection is only one of the risks that patients may be subjected to by phlebotomy (see Table 1.1). Physical injuries inflicted during the collection process can have equally serious consequences. Nerve damage, arterial nicks, lymphedema, and other injuries can be caused by those who fail to perform blood collection procedures according to the standard of care. The risk of liability for such injuries, therefore, is substantial and must be managed. (Managing this risk is covered in Chapter 7.) But the risks involved in drawing blood specimens are not limited to those that impact the health of the patient. One study showed phlebotomy to be the procedure most frequently associated with HIV exposure and that the risk of exposure is in part linked to the frequency with which healthcare professionals perform blood collection procedures (8). Twenty different diseases are known to be transmitted by blood exposure, putting those who collect and process specimens at risk of acquiring a bloodborne pathogen (9,10). Specific details on managing this risk are discussed in Chapter 8.

Proactive managers and supervisors can effectively manage all risks of phlebotomy by:

- Instituting a comprehensive phlebotomy training program
- Drafting safe phlebotomy procedures
- Implementing engineering and work-practice controls
- Maintaining high standards of performance
- Soliciting input

Instituting a Comprehensive Phlebotomy Training Program

An ad from the Birmingham Weekly offers a 40-hour training program for bartenders. Compare the consequences of mixing a drink improperly to collecting blood specimens improperly as listed in Table 1.1. How long is your training program for phlebotomists?

To minimize the risks of phlebotomy, healthcare professionals and their administrators are challenged to recognize phlebotomy for what it is—an invasive procedure with serious consequences when performed improperly—and to apply the same importance to training as they would for any other invasive procedure. Only through a comprehensive training program that teaches every aspect of phlebotomy to those who undertake the procedure can facilities and individuals ensure their own safety, the safety of their patients, the integrity of their specimens, and the preservation of the quality of care they strive to deliver.

What are the minimum training requirements for those who perform phlebotomy procedures? Unfortunately, no national standards or federal regulating agencies establish minimum phlebotomy training requirements. (See "Legislating Phlebotomy Certification," this chapter.) The Joint Commission on Accreditation of Healthcare Organizations (JCAHO) requires only that the "Hospital's leaders define the qualifications and performance expectations for all staff positions" and that "an orientation process provides initial job training and information and assess the staff's ability to fulfill specified responsibilities (11)."

Therefore, the burden of establishing a phlebotomy training program that fully addresses the risks of the procedure, that protects the patient and collector from injury, and that preserves the integrity of specimens and the quality of results extracted from those specimens belongs to employers and managers. Those who establish high standards and a comprehensive training protocol are those who most effectively manage the risk. California is the only state mandating certification for all phlebotomists.

 Tips from the Trenches: Only through a comprehensive training program that teaches every aspect of phlebotomy to those who undertake the procedure can facilities and individuals ensure their own safety, the safety of their patients, the integrity of their specimens, and the preservation of the quality of care they strive to deliver.

Because of the laboratory's expertise in specimen collection and testing, every training program must be conducted by or in concert with a laboratory representative or a healthcare professional with a strong laboratory background. When teaching blood collection procedures to non-laboratory personnel, the training program should include rotations through the laboratory department to enhance a more thorough understanding of the importance of specimen collection and processing. Every healthcare facility with specimen collection personnel should establish an in-house phlebotomy curriculum that effectively manages the risk to the patient and the collector and minimizes the employer's vulnerability to phlebotomy-related lawsuits. The list should include:

- Critical steps of the venipuncture procedure
- Proper capillary puncture procedures
- Physical risks associated with venipunctures
- Collection-related analyte alterations
- Processing-related analyte alterations
- Practices that increase risk of exposure

Even those healthcare personnel who only draw and transport specimens benefit by understanding how specimens must be processed to preserve the integrity of the specimen and ultimately the results. (See Appendix V for an outline of recommended minimum content for an in-house training curriculum. See Appendix V for resources on establishing a phlebotomy training program.)

Legislating Phlebotomy Certification

In 1999, California became the first state to enact legislation mandating that all phlebotomists be certified by a state-approved certification organization or licensed in a profession that includes phlebotomy in its official scope of practice (i.e., nurses, physicians, clinical laboratory scientists, etc.). The minimum training requirement for new phlebotomists in California now includes 40 hours of classroom instruction, 40 hours of practical instruction, and a minimum of 50 supervised punctures. This legislation sets a precedent for all healthcare professionals performing venipunctures, regardless of their discipline. Other states are considering similar legislation.

Drafting Safe Phlebotomy Procedures

Infusing the provisions of two agencies into every policy and procedure pertaining to blood specimen collection is critical to effectively managing the risks accompanying specimen collection procedures. The Clinical and Laboratory Standards Institute (formerly NCCLS) sets standards for specimen collection and handling to protect the patient from injury and negative outcomes, while the OSHA Bloodborne Pathogens Standard protects employees from accidental exposure to bloodborne pathogens.

Clinical and Laboratory Standards Institute

To manage the risk of patient injury and negative patient outcomes from the erroneous results derived from improperly performed procedures, it is critical that policies and procedures reflect the standards and guidelines established and maintained by the Clinical and Laboratory Standards Institute. These documents propose the specific details by which clinical laboratory procedures should be performed based on evidence in the literature and the expertise of nationally recognized authorities. Facilities that use Clinical and Laboratory Standards Institute documents for blood collection procedures protect patients against baseless modifications to blood collection techniques that put the patient at risk of injury and/or negative outcomes due to results altered during the collection procedure (Fig. 1.4). However, facilities can modify aspects of their procedures from those established by the Clinical and Laboratory Standards Institute to fit circumstances that may be unique to their institution, providing internal research supports such modifications. Self-styled techniques or modifications not supported in Clinical and Laboratory Standards Institute documents or established through internal studies should be avoided. Such "homemade phlebotomy" risks injury and subjects the employer to potential liability.

Homemade Phlebotomy

The following practices taught on some Internet tutorials deviate from Clinical and Laboratory Standards Institute standards and should **not** be attempted or included in a facility's procedure manual:

- If the vein has collapsed, tap the flesh above the needle with your index finger (multiple occurrences)
- Slap the site to make veins more prominent (multiple occurrences)
- It's okay to perform an arterial puncture for routine lab work (multiple occurrences)
- A discard tube is still required before a coagulation tube for routine coagulation tests (multiple occurrences)
- Incorrect order of draw (multiple occurrences)

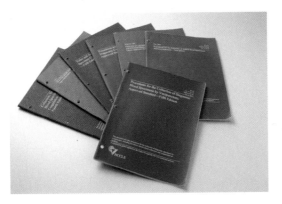

FIGURE 1.4 Standards and Guidelines published by Clinical and Laboratory Standards Institute provide a sound basis for specimen collection policies and procedures.

- Always use a winged collection set on children
- Draws above an IV are acceptable
- "Blind Sticking" is acceptable when no vein can be found
- Place the collection tray on the patient's bed
- Tourniquet goes under the armpit
- Insert the needle with the bevel down

A list of Clinical and Laboratory Standards Institute standards and guidelines that pertain to blood specimen collection is included in Appendix I.

Engineering and Work Practice Controls

Managing the risk of accidental exposure and injury cannot be effectively accomplished without fully implementing the regulations of the OSHA Bloodborne Pathogens Standard. Revised in 2001, the Standard instructs employers to implement work practice controls (i.e., policies, procedures, and practices) and engineering controls (i.e., supplies, equipment, and devices) that protect employees from injury and illness. All employers whose employees have the potential to be exposed to bloodborne pathogens are subject to OSHA guidelines. Although the standard does not apply to students, educators are well advised to voluntarily implement the guidelines for safety because the employers who hire their students will expect adherence.

The Bloodborne Pathogens Standard insists that:

- Gloves are worn during all phlebotomy procedures for diagnostic testing
- Hands are washed after gloves are removed
- Gowns or lab coats are worn whenever the risk of exposure exists
- Needles with safety features are used whenever performing a venipuncture
- Tube holder/needle assemblies are discarded as one unit immediately after use
- Food is never stored or consumed in areas in which specimens are processed, tested, or stored
- When safer devices that protect employees from bloodborne exposures become available, they must be considered annually and implemented
- Nonmanagerial employees with direct patient contact must assist in the evaluation and selection of safety devices and safe practices
- Regular inspections must be conducted to ensure devices with safety features remain functional and are used properly
- Needles must not be bent, recapped, or removed unless no alternative to disposal is feasible or if such action is required by the procedure. Justification must exist in the facility's exposure control plan supported by reliable evidence
- Sharps containers must be as close as feasible to the point of use
- All accidental needlesticks and other exposures must be recorded in the appropriate log book

The full standard is accessible at www.osha.gov.

When these and other OSHA regulations are reflected in a facility's policies and procedures, not only are employers in full compliance with federal regulations, but employees are protected to the fullest extent that written policies and procedures can provide. However, policies are only as safe as the extent to which they are enforced.

 Tips from the Trenches: Those who manage employees with blood collection responsibilities are the patient's last line of defense against poor technique and erroneous results.

Maintaining High Standards of Performance

Establishing policies and procedures based on Clinical and Laboratory Standards Institute standards and OSHA guidelines keeps facilities current in technique and compliance. However, if not reflected in actual day-to-day performance of blood collection and processing procedures, the documents painstakingly researched and drafted remain for the benefits of inspectors only. Managers who enforce the standards and guidelines reflected in their policies and procedures complete the continuity of care initiated by the Clinical and Laboratory Standards Institute and the culture of safety encouraged by OSHA (Fig. 1.5). Employees who are allowed to deviate from a facility's established procedures not only succeed in defying authority, but place the employer at risk of being held accountable for injuries and negative patient outcomes that can occur as a result of their lax enforcement of policies and procedures. To fully implement and enforce standards and guidelines reflected in one's procedure manuals, managers should:

- Include comprehensive training of your facility's policies in all new employee orientation programs
- Infuse Clinical and Laboratory Standards Institute standards of specimen collection into the training program for all employees with blood collection responsibilities

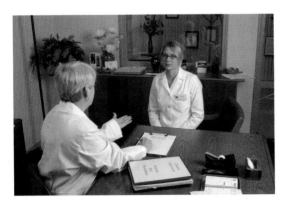

FIGURE 1.5 Managers who enforce the standards and guidelines reflected in their policies and procedures complete the continuity of care initiated by the Clinical and Laboratory Standards Institute and the culture of safety encouraged by OSHA.

- Evaluate all employees with blood collection responsibilities regularly for compliance with the facility's safety policies and blood collection procedures
- Invoke disciplinary action consistently and without fail when violations of facility policy and procedure are observed or reported
- Terminate employees who repeatedly compromise their own safety or the safety of patients

Implementing these strategies allows facilities to maintain the high standards of performance already reflected in most facilities' policies and procedures.

 Tips from the Trenches: *Employees who are allowed to deviate from a facility's established procedures not only succeed in defying authority, but place the employer at risk of being held accountable for injuries and negative patient outcomes that can occur as a result of their lax enforcement of policies and procedures.*

Recognizing that not all healthcare personnel can be taught proper blood collection technique is critical to managing the risk. For some employees, the ability to perform the procedure properly doesn't always accompany the desire. Investing additional time and patience in motivated employees may be required and is encouraged. However, it is important to recognize those employees who do not have the ability to learn proper blood collection technique and to move them into alternative positions. Likewise, recognizing employees who routinely defy prevailing safety policies and removing them from positions in which they are likely to injure themselves because of a cavalier attitude toward safety is a responsibility all managers must accept.

Those who manage employees with blood collection responsibilities manage the patient's last line of defense against poor technique and erroneous results. By implementing a comprehensive training protocol, using effective evaluation tools, and disciplining deviations from established procedures and policies, managers not only prevent injuries to employees and patients, but also help ensure that the information physicians receive and act on is accurate.

 Tips from the Trenches: *Managers who enforce the standards and guidelines reflected in their policies and procedures complete the continuity of care initiated by the Clinical and Laboratory Standards Institute and the culture of safety encouraged by OSHA.*

INSPIRING PROFESSIONALISM: STRATEGIES FOR MANAGERS

Patients' Perception of Care

Earlier in this chapter we discussed the "product" that healthcare delivers: health. How healthcare personnel can influence the patients' perception of the quality of healthcare they receive is presented in this section. Because

What Employees Want Managers to Know About Cross-Training

Once upon a time, long, long, ago, cross-training was a concept with promise. The idea was to make individuals more versatile and turn employees with limited responsibilities into ones who could perform many functions. It was efficient, it made good business sense, it was savvy, and CFOs salivated at what it might mean to the bottom line. But when hospitals started to implement the concept system-wide in the 1980s, for many it became a nightmare that would take years to awaken from.

Many employers fumbled away the golden opportunity that cross-training presented by not understanding the essentials of implementation. Lost was the trust and respect of their most valuable resource: the front-line healthcare professional. Additional casualties include the quality of care, the ability to recruit and retain dedicated employees, and that most important and fragile entity all healthcare facilities must protect: the public trust.

The ultimate objective in implementing cross-training initiatives is to reduce one's dependence on specialized employees without sacrificing the quality of care. Most administrators accomplish the former better than the latter. Poorly planned and haphazardly implemented cross-training strategies can haunt employers when they find that their new, multiskilled work force suddenly is suffering from high turnover, low morale, decreased job satisfaction, a loss of trust, and a lack of motivation.

Whether cross-training phlebotomy skills or any other function in a healthcare setting, administrators must take seriously the impact such strategies will have on the individual or risk failure. To keep such ambitious initiatives from having a negative impact on patient care and those who deliver it, consider the following seven Employee Mandates for Highly Effective Cross-Training:

Communicate—Effective cross-trainers keep us in the know. Provide full disclosure of cross-training programs at the outset and throughout the process. Give us ownership in the process by recruiting us for input on design, implementation, risk management, and negative impact issues. Give our input great weight. Nothing breeds distrust like being left out of the loop.

Educate—One of our greatest fears is the fear of the unknown. Teach us how to do something right and be thorough about it. Administrators who cut corners on our training send the signal that they don't care if it's done right. For most of us, that's an insult to our dedication and begs us to quit—or worse, quit caring.

Be Patient—Give us ample time to adjust to our expanded roles. This tells us that working within our comfort zone is critical to the process and that our acclimation to the process won't be rushed. Healthcare is serious business; we want to feel comfortable with new procedures and will not appreciate any more stress than we already have to handle.

Monitor—Assessing competency in new procedures is critical to the success of any cross- training initiative. Make sure we have all the resources we need to be trained properly.

Consider the Individual—For many of us the transition will not be welcome. Unless you are sensitive to the impact your cross-training program has on us as individuals, the collective impact it has on our morale will negate all gains.

Recruit—Telling us *why* changes are necessary makes it easier for us to buy into the concept and contribute to its success. Successful cross-training initiatives are those that give our acceptance of the concept a high priority. If we sense that our acceptance is important to you, we are more likely to work toward a successful implementation than if we think it's going to be forced upon us whether we like it or not.

Invest in Your Staff—Understand that when we have more skills to maintain, we need more continuing education opportunities. Make conferences, seminars, workshops, and in-services accessible to us and we will feel more like an important asset worthy of your investment.

(Adapted from Cross-training: mandates for managers. Phlebotomy Today 2000; 1(2). Available at www.phlebotomy.com last accessed 8/12/04.)

health is intangible, it cannot be held or physically inspected like other consumer products. Therefore, a patient's perception of the quality of the product that healthcare facilities deliver is dependent on a number of intangible elements (see Table 1.2).

Those who draw blood specimens can only influence the internal factors by collecting specimens in a manner that provides accurate results. Remember, laboratory results provide the physicians with 70% of their objective information on the patient's health status. If the specimen is collected without adherence to the proper procedure, the physician's ability to affect the patient's internal factors is compromised. However, collectors also have a significant influence on the external factors that affect the patients' perception of the quality of care they receive. Although there may be little healthcare personnel can do to improve the physical structure of the facility, making sure the phlebotomy trays they carry to the bedside and the facility's outpatient drawing areas are clean and organized contributes significantly to the patient's perception of the quality of the care the individual is capable of providing. Healthcare personnel who look healthy also give the patient confidence. When an individual's appearance reflects that their own health is a high priority, then the patient concludes that their health will be given a high priority, too. The skill of the collector also contributes significantly to the patient's trust. When venipunctures and capillary punctures are performed confidently and without incident, the patient develops a high de-

TABLE 1.2 ■ Elements Influencing a Patient's Perception of the Phlebotomy Procedure	
Internal Factors	**External Factors**
How they feel physically	The physical appearance of the facility
How they look	The health of those delivering their healthcare
The activities they are capable of performing	The skill of those delivering their healthcare
Their level of energy	Their impression of those delivering their healthcare
The absence of pain	

gree of confidence that the specimen will be processed and tested properly as well (Box 1.1).

 Tips from the Trenches: Making sure outpatient drawing areas and phlebotomy trays are clean and organized contributes significantly to the patient's perception of the quality of the care.

However, even when all of these external factors contribute to a positive impression of the quality of care the individual can provide, unprofessional behavior can undermine them all. If the collector speaks or behaves immaturely or in an unprofessional manner, his or her healthy appearance and skill in performing the procedure are discounted and can be perceived to mask a cavalier attitude toward specimen handling and testing.

A professional staff not only improves the patient's external impression of the quality of healthcare they receive, but those with a professional demeanor

---

BOX 1.1 ▇ Patient Perception

Observation: The lab coat on the person who drew my blood was clean and neat.
Perception: The laboratory must be clean and neat.

Observation: The person's scrubs were dirty and flecked with blood.
Perception: The laboratory and those who test my blood must be sloppy.

Observation: Healthcare personnel wear gloves during phlebotomy procedures.
Perception: The laboratory will process my specimen with caution and respect.

Observation: The person drawing my blood isn't wearing gloves.
Perception: They don't know much about infection control here. I wonder if this person has caught hepatitis yet. I wonder if he's passing an infection on to me.

Observation: The person who drew my blood spoke knowledgably and considerately to me.
Perception: The laboratory must be staffed with knowledgeable and considerate people.

Observation: The person who drew my blood didn't seem to know much.
Perception: The laboratory staff must not know too much about what they're doing.

Observation: The phlebotomist was pleasant and smiled often.
Perception: The laboratory must be staffed by friendly people who care about my health.

Observation: The person who drew my blood was cold and insensitive.
Perception: The laboratory must be staffed by cold and insensitive people. I wonder how that will affect how they test my blood.

Observation: The collector made sure the tubes were labeled before leaving my side.
Perception: They take specimen identification seriously here.

Observation: The collector left the room without labeling my blood.
Perception: My test results might get mixed up with someone else's.

are seen as more likely to perform blood collection procedures according to the established procedure. Therefore, it is critical on several levels for those with blood collection responsibilities to perform with professionalism if patients are to have confidence in the quality of care they are receiving.

Threats to Professionalism

Managing the risks of phlebotomy is substantially easier when one's staff is motivated to perform as professionals. Likewise, managers have a right to expect that those in patient care positions perform their duties with respect and dignity. Because of the nature of their work, healthcare personnel need and deserve to be managed with respect and dignity.

Employee morale is critical to motivate professional performance. A study conducted in 2001 showed that 13.6% of respondents ranked low morale as the number one reason they were dissatisfied with their jobs (12). A Gallop poll showed that 19% of employees are "actively disengaged" at work. Cost to employers: $292 billion to $355 billion per year (13). Low morale has many symptoms, causes, and cures. Understanding them all is the key to nurturing a professional healthcare environment.

Low morale is characterized by apathy, which can be reflected in the following behaviors:

- Calling in sick
- Coming in late
- Performing at the minimum
- Being a malcontent
- Frequent patient/co-worker complaints
- Cutting corners
- Performing half the job all the time
- High staff turnover

Employees who demonstrate these behaviors are not motivated to perform professionally. To nurture a culture of professionalism, managers must understand why employees are not motivated and provide the appropriate element to remove the barriers wherever possible. There are internal and external reasons that employees perform with apathy toward their work. Internal reasons include:

- Low self-esteem
- Inadequate reward system
- Misperception of job importance
- Misconstrued work ethic
- Resistance to change

External reasons include:

- Lack of professional work environment
- Job restructuring
- Lack of communication

To nurture professionalism, managers should attempt to understand the factors that contribute to an individual's and a staff's apathy toward professionalism and then work to provide the missing elements.

 Tips from the Trenches: Managers who recognize that they hold the key to inspiring professionalism in the workplace are more likely to inspire professionalism on many levels.

Inspiring Professionalism

Step 1: Coach Yourself First

Before evaluating what motivates your staff, perform a thorough self-evaluation of your own management style. If necessary, reform yourself to project the same behavior and disposition you expect your staff to project. Remember, managers set the example. How do you dress for work? Do you adhere to your own policies? Are you on time? Do you tell off-color jokes or use profanities in the workplace? Make sure you don't demand more of your staff or hold your employees to a higher standard than you do yourself.

Managers who recognize that they hold the key to inspiring professionalism in the workplace are more likely to inspire professionalism on many levels. Infusing strategies that inspire professional behavior into hiring practices, new employee orientation, employee evaluations, discipline, and everyday communication establishes and perpetuates a culture of professionalism. When evaluating your own contribution to the level of professionalism that exists in your staff, ask yourself these questions:

- *Do I inspire when I hire?* Weeding out applicants who you anticipate will not motivate, or be motivated by, the rest of the staff is imperative. According to one human resource expert, "ideally, a candidate should only be hired after it is determined that employer's business needs and the applicant's motivational needs are a good match (14)."
- *Do my evaluations have positive or negative undertones?* Every evaluation should discuss strengths of the employee as well as weaknesses. End each evaluation session by commenting on a positive aspect of the employee's performance, but don't make it appear obligatory. It needs to carry the employee out of the office feeling good about the experience, or at least not defeated.
- *Do I discipline fairly and consistently?* Reinforce your investment when you discipline. Offer assistance to help the employee overcome the problem. When disciplining employees, make sure every employee knows that you adhere to this management maxim: if they are worth keeping, they are worth correcting.
- *Do I inform personnel of forthcoming changes well in advance?* When instituting a change, update your staff on the progress of the change in every subsequent meeting. Talk to staff formally and informally to issue frequent reminders. Send out bulletins between meetings to update staff.

- *Do I infuse professionalism into new employee orientation?* Setting forth performance expectations during new employee orientation is something every manager knows and accomplishes. But do you establish your standards of *behavior* and *dress* up front as well? Do your new employees hear the words "our laboratory is a professional work place, and we expect new employees to act professionally" (Fig 1.6).

 Tips from the Trenches: *According to a top sales manager, "Leaders can make everyone around them better through example and wisdom or they can cultivate negativity and poor performance through their actions or inactions."(15)*

Step 2: Identify Motivators

Inspiring professional behavior requires managers to identify what motivates individuals to raise their own personal standards of performance. According to one human resources expert, "Give people what they really want most from work. The more you are able to provide what they want, the more you should expect what you really want, namely: productivity, quality, and service (16)." Perform a thorough assessment of the needs of the staff.

How do you motivate employees? You don't. You get them to motivate themselves. Instead of asking "How can I motivate these people to respect policies and procedures and to project a professional image?" ask yourself "How do I create a work environment in which employees choose to be motivated?" Don't guess at what motivates, investigate. Use informal interviews/dialogs, performance appraisals, and attitude surveys to find out what employees want most from their jobs. (A sample survey is in Appendix V.) More than likely, it's one or more of the following:

- Recognition
- Respect
- Money
- Ownership

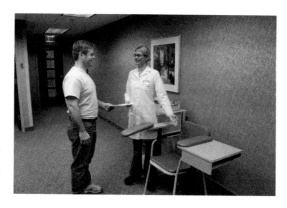

FIGURE 1.6 A patient's perception of the quality of the product that healthcare facilities deliver is dependent upon a number of intangible elements.

- Responsibility
- Appreciation
- Education
- Professional work environment

Step 3: Implement Motivators

Based on your formal or informal research, implement the motivators you have identified. Be creative and solicit the assistance of other managers, human resource staff, and phlebotomists (Fig. 1.7). It takes more time than money to implement creative strategies that motivate a staff. Be prepared to invest in dialog and creative brainstorming, and don't expect immediate results. Nurturing a culture of professionalism requires a change in perceptions for both staff and management. A staff of professionals feels that they are part of a team assembled by managers to accomplish a common goal or set of goals. For those who draw blood specimens, the goal is quality patient care through accurate results and excellent customer service. As long as the goals are accomplished, the staff needs to be recognized and rewarded with the appropriate motivators to perpetuate professionalism. If the threat of termination is the primary management motivator, the staff is less likely to feel they share a common goal with management and an "us versus them" atmosphere prevails.

Likewise, managers who sense that the staff is not engaged in the pursuit of a common goal are less apt to reward employees with the very motivators they need to make management's goals their own. If managers think of the motivators listed above as incentives instead of rewards, the downward spiral of apathy and morale begins to reverse. If employees think more outwardly toward the patient than inwardly toward dissatisfaction with management, they are more likely to be recognized as a team player.

Changing perceptions takes a long-term commitment to modifying management styles and replacing the underlying causes of apathy with the keys to motivation that you identify in your survey. Let's look at some ways in which key motivators can be provided.

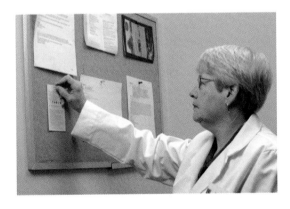

FIGURE 1.7 Informing personnel of forthcoming changes well in advance contribute to the department's morale.

Tips from the Trenches: *A staff of professionals feels that they are a part of a team assembled by managers to accomplish a common goal or set of goals. For those who draw blood specimens, the goal is quality patient care through accurate results and excellent customer service.*

Recognition and Respect

For many employees, all they want is to know that their contribution to the workplace is important and appreciated. When they know, they are inspired to raise the level of their performance, confident that their position is secure. Make it a point to tell each employee during their evaluation or right out of the blue that you know and appreciate what they bring to your facility. It can be as significant as their technical expertise or their friendly disposition with outpatients or as simple as their brilliant smile or infectious laugh. Find something in every employee and let that employee know that you recognize their gift.

Encourage those who collect specimens to seek certification. This brings recognition to them in being identified as a member of a profession and in having completed a process that has deemed them to be skilled and competent. Certification takes more effort than it does money. Most certification exams cost less than $100. Certification is a powerful tool for managers as it instills identity and pride. (See Appendix II for recommended certification organizations.)

Money

Believe it or not, money comes way down on the list of effective means of improving morale. The effects of a raise wear off soon and preexisting demotivators reemerge. Those who are employed in healthcare for its financial rewards often remain dissatisfied for other reasons.

Ownership

Everyone likes to have some say in the decisions that affect them. When a staff is invited into a process, it tells them that their input matters, which is a powerful motivator. Do you let your staff comment on proposed policy changes prior to implementing the change? Are you finding solutions to problems or inviting your staff to offer them? Even if you have the outcome already in mind, soliciting the input of employees is empowering and contributes to high morale.

Responsibility

Being put in charge of a task motivates some people. No matter how small, being given a task draws specimen collection personnel into the laboratory operations and makes them feel they are contributing on a higher level. It also tells them that you trust them enough to be given a larger role. Everyone likes to be thought of as trustworthy and valuable. This is one way to tell them.

Appreciation

How can employees give compassionate care when they feel no one is being compassionate toward them? Showing appreciation takes many forms. Complimentary meals, break snacks, promotional gifts as tokens of appreciation, etc. Don't forget the intangible forms of recognition that can be more powerful than gifts and meals. For example, saying "thank-you," "nice job," "I appreciate what you bring to the department" or recognition at informal events such as monthly meetings.

Education

When employees know that you are willing to invest in their education, it tells them that they have value. Encourage motivated phlebotomists to become certified and contribute towards the cost of certification. Invest in the staff's professional development by subscribing to learning modules, teleconferences, and online tutorials. Send selected employees to workshops and seminars. Motivated employees may welcome the opportunity to present continuing education lessons at monthly staff meetings. Recruit a pathologist to give a presentation on the importance of specimen collection. All of these activities give the impression that the employer values education and professional development.

Professional Working Environment

Do your employees realize that "street behavior" belongs on the street and that the workplace has higher standards of dress, behavior, and language? Does your facility have such standards? Do you enforce them? Do you discipline for crude language, off-color jokes, sexual innuendos, harassment, etc.? If you don't, you have a morale problem. The two go hand-in-hand.

If you are among the many employers who have let dress codes and codes of behavior slide, before enforcing an existing policy more strictly, meet with the employees and explain the policy and why it has not been enforced. Explain the problems that have arisen by lack of enforcement and why enforcement is now necessary. Make sure all employees leave the meeting knowing that they will be expected to adhere to the existing policy.

Nurturing a Culture of Customer Service

Skill and Professionalism

Customer service skills and professionalism are so closely linked that it is difficult to have one without the other. When healthcare personnel approach their role in patient care as professionals, providing excellent customer service is an extension of their persona and reflects their commitment to providing quality care to all aspects of the patient's healthcare experience. Healthcare personnel who lack professionalism often lack the motivation to make sure every encounter with every patient is positive and instills confidence that every aspect of their care is given a high priority.

Likewise, healthcare personnel who have mastered customer service skills often take a professional approach to their other responsibilities as well. They perform procedures properly, interact with co-workers with more maturity, take responsibility for their actions, function as team players, and generally contribute to a positive and professional working environment. Therefore, nurturing a culture of customer service excellence requires managers to inspire professionalism, and inspiring professionalism includes teaching customer service skills. Managers who recognize this interrelationship and promote professionalism in the workplace using the strategies detailed in the previous section find customer service skills easier to instill.

Patients' perception of the quality of care they receive is in part dependent upon two external factors: (1) the patient's impression of those delivering their healthcare and (2) the skill of those delivering their healthcare.

Nurturing a culture of customer service requires managers to ensure that those who collect specimens in the facility are properly trained and monitored. Decentralizing blood collection responsibilities from laboratory-based phlebotomists to nonlaboratory personnel makes blood collection proficiency difficult, if not impossible to maintain. Facilities that employ a decentralized phlebotomy service often find their patient satisfaction surveys plummet as the skill erodes. (See "Phlebotomy in a Multiskilled Work Force," this chapter.) Even when blood collection responsibilities are centralized in a team of phlebotomists, managers who do not properly train and regularly evaluate their staff take a self-limiting approach to customer service.

When a facility trains and maintains a staff proficient in blood collection procedures, the patients' perception of the quality of work that will be performed on their specimens can erode if they acquire a negative impression of those to whom their blood has been entrusted. Fair or not, those who draw blood specimens are the only indicators available to most patients from which to draw conclusions on how the specimen will be handled. Therefore, managers who enforce the facility's dress code policy and establish a code of conduct that reflects maturity and professionalism foster an image to the patient that invites confidence.

Code of Conduct

Managers dedicated to customer service know the power of a bad impression. Nurturing a culture of customer service excellence is difficult without establishing a code of conduct. To project a positive image to the patient and to healthcare personnel from other departments, those who collect blood specimens must know what behaviors are not acceptable. In most facilities, a code of conduct is unwritten, poorly defined, and left to speculation. As a result, street behavior can carry-over into the healthcare workplace and unintentionally threaten patients' perceptions of the quality of care their specimens receive and the accuracy of the results. Managers who draft a formal code of conduct based on facility policy define their expectations, limit the erosion of confidence, reinforce professionalism in the workplace, and nurture a culture of customer service.

 Tips from the Trenches: Nurturing a culture of customer service excellence is difficult without establishing a code of conduct.

Rewarding Customer Service Excellence

Earlier in this chapter, recognition was identified as a powerful motivator to inspire professionalism. Managers who recognize customer service skills not only reinforce the behavior in the individual, but also inspire the entire staff to emulate the recognized performance. Privately recognizing a positive customer service event by complementing the individual is important in reinforcing the level of customer service the individual provides, but public recognition inspires the bystander. When an employee or co-worker goes beyond the ordinary in providing customer service, bringing it to the attention of others announces that the level of service is valued. Post positive customer service events regularly on a department bulletin board or in a newsletter or staff update. Make mention of the event at formal or informal meetings. Bring the action to the attention of upper management in the presence of the individual. All of these forms of recognition further nurture a culture of customer service.

Scripting Techniques

One technique that many facilities use to ensure that all patients are addressed with courtesy and professionalism is called "scripting." Scripting consists of preparing a standardized script for healthcare personnel to follow when drawing specimens from every patient. It ensures that all patients are subjected to a standard and uniform interaction and that the most important components of specimen collection procedures are followed, such as proper patient identification. It also eliminates variables like attitude, interpersonal skills, and varying degrees of professionalism and helps to ensure all patients are addressed congenially and with respect. (A sample script is included in Appendix V.) Scripts consist of the following elements:

- Introduction
- Statement of purpose
- Response to inquiries
- Identify the patient
- Perform the procedure
- Thank the patient

PROFESSIONAL DEVELOPMENT AND BEHAVIOR

Personal Appearance

What does it say about the skill of a tailor whose own suit doesn't fit? Would you buy a diet book if you knew the author was 100 pounds overweight? Would you take the advice of a doctor who always looks sickly? We are walking advertisements for whatever it is we do. The image we project says a great deal about us and the quality of work we produce. Although the old saying "you can't judge a book by its cover" is true, it's human nature to draw conclusions based on whatever information we have available, however scant.

In no setting is it more important to project a positive image than in healthcare. The patients' perception of the quality of care they receive depends upon the professionalism that the staff exudes. If the phlebotomist is sloppy, patients suspect that the laboratory is sloppy as well. If the phlebotomist is cold and inconsiderate, patients suspect that the work performed on the specimen will be conducted with indifference. If the phlebotomist lacks skill, confidence, and professionalism, the patient will get the impression the specimen will not be processed or tested with integrity.

 Tips from the Trenches: *Those responsible for specimen collection must always ask themselves, "Does the image I project give the patient confidence that the blood I'm drawing will be handled properly and tested accurately?"*

Healthcare personnel who draw blood specimens must act as if they are the laboratory's ambassador. More than likely, the laboratory that tests the blood you draw does exceptional work and is staffed with highly skilled personnel dedicated to producing accurate results in a timely fashion. Patients must be able to realize that based on the way you look and interact with them. In the 5 minutes or so that it takes to address the patient and complete the procedure, the patient's impression of the quality of work conducted on the specimens is based completely and entirely on his or her impression of the collector. Most patients never see the laboratory, so the way you dress, how you're groomed, your attitude, personality, and skill all combine to give them their only impression of what the laboratory is like (see Box 1-1). Once a poor impression is imbedded, it leads patients to wonder if they are being treated and managed according to inaccurate results or results that may belong to another patient. It erodes their confidence in the facility's ability to care for them properly. (See "You Are the Lab" in the Phlebotomy Tip of the Month section of the Appendices.) Healthcare personnel who are sensitive to patients' emotions are more likely to be successful in making the phlebotomy experience uneventful. Insensitivity threatens cooperation and presents a negative impression of the facility and the integrity of the laboratory in which patients have placed this trust: that their blood will be handled with respect, tested accurately, and reported promptly.

Attitude

We only spend a few minutes with each patient, but the impact collectors can have on a patient's healthcare is phenomenal. Everyone has a bad day, but few of us carry anxiety into a patient's room that is greater than the patient's own anxiety. Because they are patients, their health is somehow threatened, and, to them, nothing else has more urgency than reclaiming their well-being. Patients need healthcare personnel to be compassionate. If we find ourselves burdened with personal issues, we should make an attempt to suppress those burdens for the short time we are interacting with those who need our help. Suppressing our own concerns long enough to care for patients is an ongoing challenge all healthcare personnel must address. (See "Dump the Baggage" in the Phlebotomy Tip of the Month section of the Appendices.)

Patients expect a great deal from us and we owe it to them to meet and exceed their expectations. The best way to do this is to treat each patient as if that patient is our best friend or a member of our family. (See "Treating All Patients As If They Were Family" in the Phlebotomy Tip of the Month section of the Appendices.) Patients have a right to quality healthcare. When it comes to phlebotomy, those rights include:

- To have their blood drawn safely
- To have their blood drawn, transported, and processed in a manner free from errors that can alter results
- To have their blood collected according to the standards
- To be properly identified
- To be treated fairly and with compassion (See Box 1.2, "Patient's Bill of Rights.")

Patients often ask healthcare personnel to perform functions beyond their usual responsibility. It's important to know which requests can be met and which must be referred to other healthcare personnel. If a patient asks for pain medication, professionalism means passing that information on to the caregiver who can shorten the time they are in pain rather than simply ignoring the request. Professionalism goes beyond mastering the mechanics of phlebotomy. It considers the entire realm of the patient (see Box 1.3: Signs of Professionalism).

Telephone Etiquette

Patients aren't the only ones who develop impressions of blood collection personnel. Anyone who phones blood collection personnel develops an image of the quality of service and work that person provides and of the department for which that individual works (Fig. 1.8). That image is also extended to the laboratory that tests the specimen. Proper telephone etiquette is essential to project a positive, professional image that instills confidence. Follow these suggestions and callers will hold you and your department in high regard:

- *Be pleasant.* Answering the phone with a pleasant voice and identifying yourself and your department to the caller is polite, professional, and tells the caller they dialed the right number. Callers who reach someone who sounds professional develop a higher opinion of that person, their department, and the quality of work both are capable of. Even if it's a department you call frequently, don't assume the person on the other end knows the sound of your voice.
- *Be ready to converse.* Few things are as annoying as answering the phone to find that the party who called you has already engaged in another conversation while waiting for you to answer. Make sure that when you place a call, you're ready to converse when the other party answers the phone.
- *Keep hold times to a minimum.* Callers don't like to wonder if they've been forgotten. If you've placed someone on hold for longer than a minute, return to the caller and ask if he or she can wait longer, or if you can call back when you have obtained the information requested.
- *End calls on a good note.* Ending a call politely leaves the caller with a good impression of you and your department. Abruptly ending a conversation without signing off is cold and tends to leave the other party wondering if he/she said something that was offensive. (See "Are Callers Glad You Answered?" in the Phlebotomy Tip of the Month section of the Appendices.)

(text continues on page 32)

BOX 1.2   Phlebotomy and the Patient's Bill of Rights

In 1971, the American Hospital Association (AHA) introduced its first version of a Patient's Bill of Rights. The current version, revised in 1992, guarantees such important rights as confidentiality and the right to refuse treatment. While federal legislation has yet to be passed, the AHA encourages healthcare institutions to tailor their proposed Bill of Rights to their own patient community by translating and/or simplifying the language as necessary. For more information on AHA's Patient Bill of Rights, visit the AHA web site at: http://www.hospitalconnect.com/aha/about/pbillofrights.html.

Many concepts proposed in the AHA Patient's Bill of Rights can be applied to phlebotomy. Although the following rights are not AHA interpretations, facilities are encouraged to apply them to their own settings.

■ Right: The patient has the right to considerate and respectful care.
Interpretation: Considerate and respectful care means knocking on the door as you enter an inpatient room and addressing all patients by Mr., Mrs., or Miss instead of "honey" or "sugar;" it means saying "please" and "thank-you;" it means stopping short of the pulled curtain and asking for permission to enter before barging in, and it means being gentle. It also means removing the needle when patients are in agony, and knowing when to quit.

■ Right: The patient has the right to, and is encouraged to obtain from physicians and other direct caregivers, relevant, current, and understandable information concerning diagnosis, treatment, and prognosis.
Interpretation: Phlebotomists are not in a position to discuss the management, diagnosis, or prognosis of any patient, nor should they make assumptions based on the tests ordered. Although this right states that patients are entitled to such information, most specimen collection personnel simply don't have access to the information necessary to counsel patients. Instead, defer such requests to the patient's nurse or physician as appropriate.

■ Right: The patient is entitled to the opportunity to discuss and request information related to the specific procedures and/or treatments.
Interpretation: Are specimen collection personnel obligated to tell the patient what tests are being drawn? Every facility has its own policy on this issue, so it's best to follow facility protocol. If the facility allows personnel to reveal the tests being ordered, is the collector obligated to explain what the tests test for? Again, all facilities draw the line differently. Few who draw blood specimens can speak with authority on the nature of all laboratory tests. Therefore, such explanations are a function not only of facility policy, but also the collector's technical expertise. The Bill doesn't say who is obligated to discuss specific procedures, only that the patient has the right to request information. Only those authorized should respond to such requests.

■ Right: The patient is entitled to the opportunity to discuss and request information related to the risks involved with specific procedures and/or treatments.
Interpretation: How many phlebotomists tell patients that phlebotomy poses the risks of nerve injury, arterial hemorrhage, and the transfusion of incompatible blood due to patient misidentification? Probably none. Yet all these are risks of the procedure. Remember, the Bill of Rights says patients have the right to request information, but it doesn't indicate the information should be presented before every medical procedure. Walking down the hall

has risks. In fact, hospitalization is the eighth leading cause of death in the United States (due to nosocomial infections, medication errors, etc.), but we don't advise patients of every complication, especially those that occur rarely. Nevertheless, when asked, patients should be notified of the risks of phlebotomy according to facility protocol.

■ Right: Patients have the right to know when those involved are students, residents, or other trainees.

Interpretation: Phlebotomists in training and under the direct supervision of a seasoned phlebotomist should inform the lucid patient that the individual is new to the procedure. For patients who are sedated or otherwise unconscious, the facility should establish its own protocol. Not everyone likes to have blood drawn by novices who are not yet cleared to draw blood unsupervised. Allowing them to opt out respects their right to know and is good customer service.

■ Right: The patient has the right to refuse a recommended treatment or plan of care to the extent permitted by law and hospital policy and to be informed of the medical consequences of this action.

Interpretation: Patients have the right to refuse to be drawn for a blood test. Of course, specimen collection personnel should attempt to explain how the procedure contributes to their overall care in general terms if it is perceived that the patient may lack the proper information to rationally refuse. However, as stated above, the information provided should be general in nature and should not delve into diagnosis, prognosis, or constitute medical advice or counseling. Handling refusals from children or patients with impaired mental status should be handled according to facility protocol.

■ Right: The patient has the right to every consideration of privacy.

Interpretation: Where appropriate and possible, phlebotomists should be mindful that others within view and within earshot don't have a right to see and hear what's going on with other patients. This is especially important in drawing areas in which barriers to sight and sound are not physically possible. Remember, you are being watched and overheard all the time.

■ Right: The patient has the right to expect that all communications and records pertaining to his/her care will be treated as confidential by the hospital.

Interpretation: This means that comments specific to a patient's confidential information should not be made where others not privy to the information can overhear. This is not limited to the ears of other patients or visitors, but to those of coworkers and employees from other departments as well. The same holds true for reports and documents. With the implementation of HIPPA guidelines, phlebotomists are significantly more alert to patient confidentiality breaches than ever before.

■ Right: The patient has the right to review the records pertaining to his/her medical care and to have the information explained or interpreted as necessary, except when restricted by law.

Interpretation: Although patients have the right to review their charts, it is inappropriate for phlebotomists to make them available. Requests from patients should be forwarded to the patient's nurse or physician. Should a patient ask the individual collecting the specimen to interpret a laboratory result, the patient should be referred to the physician who ordered the test so that he/she can put the result in the proper context for the patient. Because phlebotomists don't have a full perspective of the patient's condition, information given out of context can be misleading, even disturbing, to the patient.

BOX 1.3   Signs of Professionalism

Outward Signs of Professionalism

- Scrubs or lab coats are clean and without excessive wear
- Not wearing jeans, tank tops, or street clothes or dressing immodestly
- Hair is well groomed without extreme styling or unnatural coloring
- No excessive jewelry, piercing, or tattoos
- Hands are clean and fingernails are trimmed short without flamboyant polish
- Name tag is neat and visible
- Make-up applied conservatively
- Perfume or aftershave is not excessive
- Breath is not offensive
- General appearance represents physical well-being

Behaviors That Project Professionalism

- Knocking on inpatient doors while entering
- Asking permission before entering a closed-curtain area
- Introducing yourself and stating your purpose
- Smiling
- Making eye contact
- Speaking clearly
- Listening with compassion
- Explaining the procedure to those who require it (e.g., children)
- Investing time in calming fears
- Responding to patient requests (within the limits of facility policy)
- Discarding dropped supplies and equipment
- Respecting patient refusals with composure
- Respecting patient requests to return at a later time whenever possible
- Respecting patient privacy and confidentiality
- Resisting the temptation to tell off-color jokes, use foul language, make sexual innuendos, or to laugh with those who do

Telephone Etiquette That Projects Professionalism

- Answering the phone with courtesy and kindness in your voice
- Identifying yourself and your department whenever placing or receiving a call
- Keeping callers on hold no longer than 1 minute
- Being ready to converse when the other party answers
- Answering the phone within three rings
- Ending all calls with "Thank-you. Goodbye."

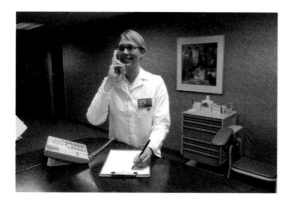

FIGURE 1.8 Anyone who phones blood collection personnel develops an image of the quality of service and work that person provides and the department for which that individual works.

Certification, Education, and Professional Affiliation

Nothing inspires professionalism like being certified in one's profession. Certification brings pride in having completed a process that deems one to be skilled and competent. Phlebotomy certification takes more effort than it does money. Most certification exams are less than $100. Certification offers the following:

- Gives a person identity and a sense of belonging
- Recognizes one's skills and expertise
- Improves one's self-image
- Identifies an individual as being skilled and competent

Make sure the certification you obtain is meaningful. Some agencies offer "certification" based on attending a weekend phlebotomy course or simply providing documentation of prior work experience in phlebotomy. Make sure the certification you seek at least involves taking an exam. Certification is legislated in California, Nevada, and Louisiana. In all other states, certification is up to the individual or the facility. For a list of recommended certification organizations and their requirements, see Appendix II.

Professionals constantly seek ways to continue their education. Examples of continuing education opportunities include:

- Subscribe to learning modules, teleconferences, online tutorials, etc.
- Attend workshops/seminars and share the information with co-workers upon your return
- Present a continuing education lesson at a monthly staff meeting
- Solicit a laboratory director, medical director, or pathologist to give a presentation on the importance of specimen collection

A list of organizations offering continuing education opportunities is listed in Appendix III.

Finally, become involved in a professional membership organization. Professional affiliation contributes to a culture of professionalism by inspiring members to excel and become active in the growth and improvement of themselves and the organization. Become active in conference development;

volunteer for offices or committee positions in the organization; promote the organization with your peers. Several organizations welcome those with phlebotomy responsibilities or interests. See Box 1.4 for a complete listing.

 Tips from the Trenches: Professional affiliation inspires healthcare personnel to excel and become active in the growth and improvement of themselves and their organization.

Patient Courtesies

How we address patients says a great deal about our degree of professionalism. Most healthcare professionals know that people have apprehensions about invasive procedures, even those as simple as a venipuncture. For many patients, allaying the fear of phlebotomy can be difficult. Because patient apprehension is impossible to predict, it is best that healthcare personnel approach each patient as if the procedure brings great anxiety (see "Needle Phobia," Chapter 4).

To respond with professionalism to the needs of the inpatient population, it's important to look at hospitalization from a patient's perspective. Upon admission, patients are ushered into unfamiliar surroundings and stripped of their personal effects and basic liberties. Wallets, purses, jewelry, clothing, privacy, dignity, and the power over what happens to them are removed and not returned until they are released. They're inspected, examined, prodded, probed, and questioned on the most intimate details of their personal lives. They are given embarrassing garments to wear and denied most of the freedoms they took for granted in the outside world—sometimes even the freedom to get out of bed without permission. A multitude of strange faces comes and goes, each with a mandated interest in their bodies or bodily functions that if pursued anywhere outside of a healthcare setting would be an insulting invasion of privacy.

To the patient, healthcare personnel who are attuned to the potential for patients to feel "institutionalized" can be a refreshing exception to an overly

---

BOX 1.4 Membership Organizations for Those with Blood Specimen Collection Responsibilities

American Medical Technologists (AMT). 710 Higgins Road, Park Ridge, IL 60068. 847-823-5169 or 800-275-1268. www.amt1.org

American Society for Clinical Laboratory Science (ASCLS). 6701 Democracy Boulevard, Suite 300, Bethesda, MD 20817. 301-657-2768. www.ascls.org; ascls@ascls.org

American Society for Clinical Pathology (ASCP). 2100 West Harrison Street, Chicago, IL 60612. 312-738-1336. www.ascp.org; Info@ascp.org

Clinical Laboratory Management Association (CLMA). 989 Old Eagle School Road, Suite 815, Wayne PA 19087. 610-995-9580. www.clma.org; support@clma.org

insensitive staff. For children, hospitalization is especially traumatic. (See Chapter 4 for strategies on calming the fears of pediatric patients.)

When healthcare personnel knock on the patient's door on their way into the room, it shows a respect for the few square feet to which the patient has been assigned. (Those who interact with the patient many times in the course of the day may find this courtesy to be awkwardly repetitive and unnecessary and should take advantage of other opportunities to show respect for the patient's privacy and dignity.)

If the curtain is pulled, ask permission to enter so as not to embarrass the patient who may be using a bedpan, urinal, or bedside commode or to interrupt a patient's confidential conversation with his or her physician or clergy member. If the blood draw is not urgent, offering to come back later shows the patient that you respect their privacy.

Likewise, if the patient is in the middle of a meal, offer to return after they have finished unless the time of draw has urgency. Those with good customer service skills allow themselves to be inconvenienced.

Professional behavior requires healthcare personnel to leave the room the same way they find it (Fig. 1.9). If you moved the bedside tray out of your way, move it back so that the patient's belongings are once again within reach. If you lowered the bedrail, return it to its upright position. Make sure the call light remains accessible.

Regardless of the setting, those who are new to the patient should begin by identifying themselves and their purpose. Those who have already established a rapport with the patient need only identify their purpose. An attempt should be made to arouse patients who appear asleep or sedated. Avoid calling patients by pet names such as "honey" or "sugar." It may be your nature to use such terms of endearment with strangers, but it's unprofessional in a healthcare setting, and not all patients will appreciate it. Instead, use more respectful terms such as Mr., Ms., sir, or ma'am, unless the patient gives you permission to be less formal.

If the patient expresses an interest in knowing the nature of the tests that are to be drawn, healthcare professionals should explain them in layman's terms. If the patient presses for further information or if you are unsure of

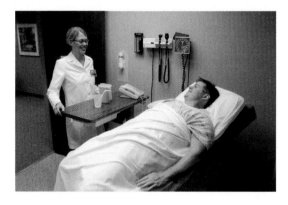

FIGURE 1.9 Professional behavior requires healthcare personnel to leave the room the same way they find it.

the nature of the test(s), refer the patient to the nurse or ordering physician for clarification. If the patient verbalizes or demonstrates an apprehension about the procedure, it may be prudent to explain the steps of the procedure as described in Chapter 4 before performing the puncture. Once the procedure begins, distracting attention from the procedure with casual conversation can serve to calm the anxious patient.

Professionals recognize that patients have the right to refuse any procedure, including phlebotomy (see Box 1.2 "Patient's Bill of Rights"). Patients may refuse a blood draw for many reasons.

- Sometimes "no" means "I don't understand why this blood test is important to my care." If so, a simple explanation that puts the procedure into perspective is all that is necessary. But be careful not to get too detailed or technical; you may entrench their resistance even further.
- Sometimes "no" means "not right now." Perhaps the patient just received bad news, or a visitor who just left said something upsetting. Maybe their dinner tray just arrived and they don't want it to get cold. If you sense their apprehension is just for the moment, offer to come back in a little while. Showing that you are flexible enough to return may be all they need to know in order to become cooperative later.
- Sometimes "no" means "I need to exert some authority over someone." While they are hospitalized, patients do nothing except take orders from strangers. Swallow this, eat that, come with me, stay in bed, wake up, go to sleep, etc. For those who are used to giving orders, being told what to do and when to do it can be difficult. Healthcare personnel who realize when a patient needs to demonstrate some authority over what happens to them by refusing a blood test are in a good position to gain the respect of that patient by politely complying unless the phlebotomy has urgency. If you can come back later, you may find the patient much more cooperative.
- Sometimes "no" comes from family members who have become distraught over the care of the patient or who recognize that the patient is in the last moments of life. Healthcare personnel must be especially sensitive to the needs of family members and respect their refusal politely and compassionately.
- Sometimes "no" simply means "no." Professionals recognize when diplomacy is a lost cause and respectfully dismiss themselves without further provocation.

Professionals don't take refusals personally, but respond with composure, explaining the importance of the tests to the physician's management of the patient's care. Professionals are acutely aware that hospitalization can be viewed by some patients as institutionalizing and are sensitive to patients who become distraught. Proceeding with a venipuncture after a rational refusal may lead to a complaint against the phlebotomist or even prompt a charge of battery. Therefore, it's important for healthcare personnel to know when to reason with the difficult patient and when to politely withdraw. When refusals are final, notify the nurse or immediate caregiver in charge of the patient. Because these individuals have an established rapport with their patients, they may be able to gain their cooperation. When patients are unwavering, have their immediate caregiver document the refusal in the patient's chart.

Granting patients these courtesies and considerations restores an element of dignity to patients and can make the difference between a positive and negative phlebotomy experience for the patients and you. Healthcare personnel who show respect for patients will find them to be more cooperative for venipunctures and less likely to be frustrated should a second attempt to obtain blood become necessary.

REFERENCES

1. Cortizas M. The risks associated with phlebotomy decentralization. *Lab Notes* 1997;7:1,4.
2. Q&A. *Cap Today* 2002;6:114.
3. Nelson K. Recentralizing phlebotomy services in the clinical lab. *Adv Med Lab Prof* 2002; 14:21–24.
4. Berger D. Direct-to-consumer testing [Editorial]. *MLO* 2000;32:6.
5. Becan-McBride K. Preanalytical phase and important requisite of laboratory testing. *Adv Med Lab Prof* 1998:12–17.
6. Dale J. Preanalytic variables in laboratory testing. *Lab Med* 1998;29:540–545.
7. Paxton A. Stamping out specimen collection errors. *CAP Today* 1999;13(5):1,14–16,18.
8. Jagger J. Risky procedure, risky devices, risky job. *Adv Exposure Prev* 1994;1:4–9.
9. Jagger J. Rates of needlestick injury caused by various devices in a university hospital. *N Engl J Med* 1988; 319(5):284–8.
10. Godin G, Naccache H, Morel S, et al. Determinants of nurses' adherence to universal precautions for venipunctures. *AJIC* 2000;28:359–364.
11. Joint Commission: CAMH. *Comprehensive accreditation manual for hospitals.* Oakbrook Terrace, IL: Joint Commission on Accreditation of Healthcare Organizations, 2000:HR-4.
12. Staff morale low? Before spending money, hear what employees want. *Same-Day Surgery* (online). July, 2002, www.ahcpub.com/ahc_root_html/hot/articles/sds072002. html (accessed 4/6/03).
13. Heathfield S. Set them free: two musts for motivation. What You Need To Know About Human Resources. http://humanresources.about.com/library/weekly/aa032801a.htm (accessed 4/6/03).
14. Foster, M. Employee satisfaction: the healthcare success factor. Available at www. ikidney.com (accessed 1/13/05).
15. Lauer C. Make your workers the stars. Modern Healthcare. Available at www. modernhealthcare.com (accessed 4/2/03).
16. Motivating your staff in a time of change. What you need to know about human resources. http://humanresources.about.com/library/weekly/nosearch/nuc021503a.htm (accessed 4/6/03).

REVIEW QUESTIONS

1. Creating phlebotomy positions in the 1970s allowed the higher paid laboratory technologists to concentrate on:
   a. blood specimen collection
   b. phlebotomy supervision
   c. the testing phase of clinical laboratory work
   d. unionization

2. In the 1980s, patient satisfaction surveys began to show that the more employees a patient encountered:
   a. the more satisfied they were with their care
   b. the less satisfied they were with their care
   c. the more expensive it was to treat them
   d. the longer their length of stay became

3. As healthcare delivery systems expanded in the 1980s, it became increasingly obvious to administrators that:
   a. employing individuals who have only one skill was an inefficient use of human resources
   b. phlebotomists were an integral part of the laboratory staff
   c. cross-training phlebotomists was costly and inefficient
   d. nursing assistants were overutilized

4. Efficiencies gained in the decentralization of phlebotomists were lost by:
   a. the unionization of healthcare
   b. the growth of HMOs
   c. delays in testing and the cost of recollections
   d. increased salaries for cross-trained personnel

5. Up to ____ % of the errors that can alter test results occur during the "preanalytical" phase.
   a. 13
   b. 46
   c. 56
   d. 85

6. Procedures pertaining to blood specimen collection should be based on documents issued by:
   a. OSHA and the Clinical and Laboratory Standards Institute
   b. FDA and OHSA
   c. JCAHO and Clinical and Laboratory Standards Institute
   d. CAP and NSI

7. Which state became the first state to enact legislation mandating that all phlebotomists be certified?
   a. Louisiana
   b. New York
   c. Michigan
   d. California

8. A study conducted in 2001 showed that _____ % of respondents ranked low morale as the number one reason they were dissatisfied with their jobs.
   a. 15.4
   b. 13.6
   c. 56
   d. 12
9. Managers foster an image to the patient that invites confidence when they:
   a. establish a code of conduct
   b. consistently discipline
   c. fairly compensate employees
   d. draft policies that reflect OSHA guidelines
10. Outward signs of professionalism include:
   a. recognizing one's importance to patient care
   b. hair that is well groomed without extreme styling or unnatural coloring
   c. excessive body art
   d. concealed employee identification badge
11. Telephone etiquette that projects professionalism includes:
   a. referring to callers as "honey" or other terms of endearment
   b. keeping callers on hold longer than 1 minute
   c. answering the phone after 3 rings
   d. identifying yourself and your department whenever placing or receiving a call
12. Healthcare personnel who are asked by patients to perform functions that are not their responsibility should:
   a. accommodate the patient's request as providing good customer service
   b. ignore the patient's request
   c. bring the request to the attention of the patient's immediate caregiver
   d. document the request in the patient's chart.

Selecting and Assembling Equipment

2

KEY TERMS AND DEFINITIONS

Hemolysis The rupture of red blood cells (RBCs) during collection, handling, storage, or transportation, resulting in contamination and tingeing of the serum or plasma with the hemoglobin pigment.

Plasma The liquid portion of the blood after centrifugation of a specimen in which an anticoagulant has prevented clot formation.

Serum The liquid portion of the blood after centrifugation of a specimen that is allowed to clot.

INTRODUCTION

Along with professionalism and good technique, successful specimen collection depends on selecting the proper equipment according to each patient's unique set of variables. This chapter discusses making appropriate equipment selections to ensure the procedure is performed properly and professionally. Topics include test orders, supplies and equipment, and equipment assembly. After reading this chapter, the reader should be able to:

- Select venipuncture equipment appropriate for the vein selected and tests ordered
- List the additives in the most commonly used specimen collection tubes
- Discuss the advantages using a tube holder has over a syringe assembly when performing venipunctures
- State the appropriate use of the various sizes of needles available for phlebotomy

TEST ORDERS

In most states, blood tests must be ordered and signed by a physician, nurse practitioner, or other qualified medical professional. Laboratory tests usually are ordered in writing on the patient's chart or on a prescription pad or approved order form from the physician's office. Should the physician verbally order a test for an inpatient, the order must be documented on the patient's chart and later signed by the ordering practitioner. However, in emergencies where the patient's life is in danger, there is not always time to secure the physician's permission. Therefore, whenever healthcare personnel order tests in anticipation of the physician's approval, the healthcare professional must have the authority to place the order, and the order must be written in the patient's chart and eventually approved by the physician by signature. For outpatients, verbal orders must be followed by a written order signed by the physician. Accreditation and certifying agencies can cite facilities that charge for tests without signed orders. Some states, however, allow patients to order their own lab tests. (See "Direct Access Testing," this chapter.)

When outpatients arrive at the facility or drawing station for specimen collection, their test orders are transcribed manually or electronically onto requisitions that contain complete patient and test information by a patient registration clerk or the specimen collection personnel. Requisitions may be preprinted forms with the test(s) requested checked or handwritten or as computer-generated preprinted labels. For inpatients, requisitions are prepared by ward clerks, unit secretaries, nurses, or other caregivers designated to convert physician orders into test requisitions. Collection personnel can be notified by phone or through the hospital information system (HIS) interfaced with the laboratory information system (LIS).

Test requisitions must contain the following information:

- Patient's first and last name with middle initial
- Ordering physician's name
- Patient's unique identification (i.e., medical record) number
- Patient's date of birth
- Patient's location if inpatient (i.e., room number and bed)
- Test(s) to be performed
- Billing information if outpatient (i.e., ICD-9 codes, diagnosis, etc.)
- Testing requirements (e.g., fasting, stat, timed, etc.)

Specimen collection personnel should review the test requisition for errors, completeness, and the test(s) requested. In addition, they should correct any errors or duplicate orders, investigate any information that requires clarification or confirmation, and review the tests for any special requirements the test or physician may have. Examples include:

- Fasting or dietary restrictions
- Timed orders
- Patient posture requirements (e.g., recumbent)
- Timing the draw around patient medication dosage or administration
- Ingestion of a meal or measured glucose (e.g., 2-hour postprandial glucose, glucose tolerance tests, etc.)

After obtaining all pertinent information and assuring all test requirements are met, collection personnel then proceed to the next step in the collection process: patient identification and specimen collection.

Tips from the Trenches: Specimen collection personnel should review the test requisition for errors, completeness, and the test(s) requested.

Direct Access Testing

More states are enacting legislation allowing patients to order their own blood tests. So-called "direct access testing" allows patients to enter any hospital offering the service, request a lab test or series of tests, and receive results directly. Approval by the patient's physician is not necessary. (Insurance typically does not cover patient-ordered testing since most policies require a physician's order.) For patients who are frustrated by the many "gatekeepers" of healthcare, the freedom to order one's own laboratory tests is a significant step toward managing their own health. Although such legislation is controversial, many laboratories are providing the service to their patient population to provide an additional service to the community and enhance revenues. However, opponents argue that patients aren't trained to properly interpret test results and may mismanage their own health. Some fear that direct access testing means fewer physician office visits and decreased revenues. Nevertheless, the luxury of ordering one's own lab tests and receiving the results directly is changing healthcare and impacting on those who draw blood specimens.

Currently, 18 states allow patients to order their own lab tests and 34 states prohibit the practice. In the states that allow it, the menu of allowable tests varies substantially. Colorado, for example, does not limit the tests its citizens can order for themselves, whereas Maryland limits patients to ordering cholesterol testing only.

Table 2.1 is a list of those states that offer direct access testing at the time of publication.

SUPPLIES AND EQUIPMENT

Those with blood collection responsibilities should have a wide variety of collection supplies and equipment readily accessible. A fully stocked phlebotomy tray or table keeps supplies organized and should include all materials required to perform the procedure and those supplies necessary to react to potential complications. The most common supplies are (Fig. 2.1):

- Tourniquet
- Gauze
- Alcohol prep
- Nonlatex gloves
- Needles of various lengths and gauges
- Tube holder adapters
- Syringes

(text continues on page 47)

TABLE 2.1 ■ Summary of Direct Access Testing by State

State	Direct Access Testing Permitted	Limitations on Direct Access Testing (DAT)	Notes
Alabama	No	DAT prohibited	
Alaska	Yes	No limits	State law doesn't prohibit direct access testing
Arizona	No	DAT prohibited	
Arkansas	Yes	See Notes	Hospital laboratories may not perform direct access testing, but other laboratories are not similarly restricted
California	Yes	Limited	California currently allows glucose, cholesterol, pregnancy, occult blood, and HIV (FDA-approved home collection kit only) to be provided via direct access testing. Beginning January 1, 2002, the state also allowed all tests approved by the US Food and Drug Administration for over-the-counter use without a prescription to be provided as direct access tests
Colorado	Yes	No limits	State law doesn't prohibit direct access testing
Connecticut	No	DAT prohibited	
Delaware	Yes	No limits	State law doesn't prohibit direct access testing
District of Columbia	Yes	No limits	State law doesn't prohibit direct access testing
Florida	No	DAT prohibited	State law does allow use of FDA-approved home-based HIV collection kits
Georgia	No	DAT prohibited	
Hawaii	No	DAT prohibited	
Idaho	No	DAT prohibited	
Illinois	Yes	Limited	Only tests classified as waived under the federal Clinical Laboratory Improvement Amendments (CLIA) of 1988 may be self-authorized
Indiana	Yes	No limits	State law doesn't prohibit direct access testing
Iowa	No	DAT prohibited	
Kansas	Yes	No limits	While Kansas does not prohibit direct access testing, hospital laboratories are required to specify who may authorize laboratory testing
Kentucky	No	DAT prohibited	
Louisiana	Yes	No limits	State law doesn't prohibit direct access testing
Maine	Yes	Limited	Maine allows self-authorization for glucose (provided the individual is a diagnosed diabetic), cholesterol (total and HDL), urine pregnancy, and fecal occult blood

TABLE 2.1 ■ Summary of Direct Access Testing by State (continued)

State	Direct Access Testing Permitted	Limitations on Direct Access Testing (DAT)	Notes
Maryland	Yes	Limited	Maryland allows direct access testing for cholesterol (total cholesterol and HDL only). The laboratory must be licensed to perform testing if it provides testing services without a medical order
Massachusetts	No	DAT prohibited	
Michigan	Yes	Limited	Only tests classified as waived under CLIA may be self-authorized
Minnesota	Yes	No limits	State law doesn't prohibit direct access testing
Mississippi	Yes	Hospitals: DAT prohibited. Other Laboratories: No limits	Hospital-based laboratories may not perform direct access testing, but state law does not prohibit other laboratories from performing direct access testing
Missouri	Yes	Limited	Hospitals may not perform direct access testing on inpatients. Otherwise, there are no restrictions on the types of tests that may be performed via direct access
Montana	Yes	No limits	State law doesn't prohibit direct access testing
Nebraska	Yes	No limits	State law doesn't prohibit direct access testing
Nevada	Yes	Limited	Nevada permits direct access testing only in cases where the test may be performed with a testing device or kit approved by the FDA for use in the home that is available to the public without a prescription
New Hampshire	Yes	No limits	State law doesn't prohibit direct access testing
New Jersey	Yes	Limited	Only tests classified as waived under CLIA may be self-authorized
New Mexico	Yes	No limits	State law doesn't prohibit direct access testing
New York	Yes	Limited	Only ABO blood grouping and Rh typing may be provided as direct access testing
North Carolina	No	DAT prohibited	
North Dakota	No	DAT prohibited	
Ohio	Yes	No limits	State law does not prohibit direct access testing; however laboratory must be state certified if performing testing for sexually transmitted diseases
Oklahoma	Yes	No limits	State law doesn't prohibit direct access testing
Oregon	No	DAT prohibited	
Pennsylvania	No	DAT prohibited	

(continues)

TABLE 2.1 ■ Summary of Direct Access Testing by State *(continued)*			
State	**Direct Access Testing Permitted**	**Limitations on Direct Access Testing (DAT)**	**Notes**
Puerto Rico	Yes	Limited	Puerto Rico does not allow hospitals to perform direct access testing, but independent laboratories may perform via direct access those laboratory tests that are approved by the federal Food and Drug Administration for over-the-counter use
Rhode Island	No	DAT prohibited	
South Carolina	No	DAT prohibited	
South Dakota	Yes	No limits	State law doesn't prohibit direct access testing
Tennessee	No	DAT prohibited	
Texas	Yes	No limits	State law doesn't prohibit direct access testing
Utah	Yes	Limited	State law limits direct access testing performed at hospital-based laboratories to those tests that can be understood by the patient. It is unclear whether this restriction applies to other laboratories
Vermont	Yes	No limits	State law doesn't prohibit direct access testing
Virginia	Yes	No limits	State law doesn't prohibit direct access testing
Washington	Yes	No limits	
West Virginia	Yes	No limits	State law does not prohibit direct access testing; however, HIV testing may require physician's order
Wisconsin	Yes	No limits	State law doesn't prohibit direct access testing
Wyoming	No	DAT prohibited	

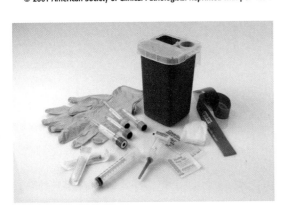

FIGURE 2.1 Healthcare professionals with blood collection responsibilities should have a wide variety of collection supplies and equipment accessible at the patient's side.

- Winged collection sets
- Collection tubes of various sizes, with and without additives
- Capillary collection tubes with and without additives
- Adhesive bandages, preferably hypoallergenic
- Sharps container
- Waste receptacle
- Iodine or chlorhexidine disinfectants for blood culture collections
- Safety transfer devices
- Marking pen

Supplies should always be kept within reach. Should more gauze or tubes be needed during the procedure, reaching for supplies not within arm's length puts the patient at risk of injury. It is important, however, not to place supplies on the patient's bed where they are likely to be swept off by sudden movements. Also avoid placing phlebotomy trays on the patient's bedside tray. The bottom of the phlebotomy tray likely contains a host of pathogenic microorganisms. Placing collection trays on the same table that the patient eats from, leans on, and places his/her personal belongings on (eyeglasses, hearing aids, dentures, etc.) eventually exposes the patient to a multitude of potentially infectious bacteria. Instead, put the tray on a chair or other elevated stand that can be pulled within reach. (See "Bug Bombs" in the Phlebotomy Tip of the Month Section of the Appendices.)

 Tips from the Trenches: *Dropped supplies or equipment should never be used on a patient even if sterility has not been compromised. When healthcare personnel pick up fallen objects from the floor and use them for the venipuncture, the perception to the patient is that the collector used contaminated supplies or equipment during the puncture. Should a tube holder, tourniquet, tube, etc. fall, let the patient see you discard it. Keeping extra supplies within reach prevents this disturbing perception and retains patient confidence.*

It Could Happen to You

A nurse successfully obtained blood from an emergency room patient, but had positioned her supplies out of reach. With the needle still in the patient's arm, she had to stretch awkwardly to retrieve the gauze pad so she could apply pressure when the needle was removed. By so doing, she drove the needle deeper into the patient's arm inflicting a permanent and disabling nerve injury.

Question: What could have been done to prevent this injury?

Answer: If the nurse had kept the specimen collection supplies within reach, she would not have put the patient at risk by stretching to retrieve the gauze and the needle would likely have remained stationary. Keeping supplies within reach at all times prevents situations that can cause the needle to pierce or lacerate vulnerable structures beneath the skin.

Tubes and Additives

A wide variety of specimen collection tubes are available for the multitude of tests that can be required to be performed on patient blood. Most tubes contain an additive to either prevent or promote clotting of the specimen. These additives are manufactured and added to tubes under very exacting specifications and can significantly alter test results if the tube is not properly filled or handled during and after collection. Healthcare personnel with specimen collection responsibilities must be aware of the nature of these additives and their affect on the blood in order to collect specimens that are not altered during the collection process. Because it is impossible to detect many specimen collection errors after the specimen is collected, those who underestimate the role additives play in the quality of the specimen can contribute to erroneous results and patient mismanagement. Therefore, it is critical to the patient that collectors use proper technique and collect specimens according to facility policy based on tube manufacturer's instructions and Clinical and Laboratory Standards Institute (formerly NCCLS) standards (Box 2.1).

Table 2.2 lists the most common additives, their function, use, and limitations.

Sodium Citrate Tube–Blue Stopper

Sodium citrate removes calcium from the coagulation cascade. Without calcium, clot formation cannot occur. This additive is used to prepare specimens for coagulation studies such as prothrombin time (PT), activated partial thromboplastin time (aPTT), and special factor assays such as factor VIII and factor IX. The amount of anticoagulant in the tubes is calculated by manufacturers to provide a 9:1 blood:anticoagulant ratio, which is necessary for accurate results. Therefore, it is critical that these tubes be filled to at least 90% of their stated capacity to maintain the ratio. Because liquid sodium citrate is so sensitive to deviations from the optimum fill, any fill

---

BOX 2.1   Tube Handling Errors That Corrupt Specimens and Cause Erroneous Results

- Manually pouring or transferring the contents of one tube into another
- Vigorously mixing tubes
- Filling tubes in the incorrect order of draw
- Manually removing additive prior to filling the tube*
- Removing a clot from a tube containing an anticoagulant and submitting the specimen for testing
- Underfilling a tube containing an anticoagulant
- Overfilling tubes containing additives

- Failing to invert tubes immediately upon filling
- Collecting specimens in the wrong tube (e.g., lithium level collected into lithium heparin tube)

*Except when drawing PT or aPTT levels on patients with a hematocrit greater than 55%.

greiner bio-one

GREINER BIO ONE VACUETTE® CAPS	Additive	Number of Inversions per NCCLS	Remarks	Old Tube
	109M (3.2%) Sodium Citrate	4	**Coagulation Tests** Follow your institution's guidelines for specimen transport and processing.	
	Clot Activator Gel Serum Separator **NOTE**	5-10	**Serum Chemistry Profiles** **Clot activator should be mixed by inverting the specimen which facilitates complete clotting. **	
	Lithium Heparin Lithium Heparin Gel Sodium Heparin	5-10	**Plasma Chemistry Profiles** Lithium Heparin prevents clotting by tube inversions.	
	K_3EDTA K_2EDTA	8-10	EDTA for whole blood hematology determinations and Immunohematology testing (ABO, Rh typing, antibody screens, etc.)	
	K_2EDTA Gel	8-10	**PCR Assays** i.e., HIV and HCV viral loads	
	Potassium Oxalate Sodium Fluoride	5-10	Glucose Testing	
	Sodium Heparin Non-Additive	5-10	Trace Element Lead Testing	

● yellow - Gel Separation   ● black - Standard Draw   ● white - Pediatric Draw

For further assistance please contact Greiner Bio-One at 888 286 3883 or email to info@us.vacuette.com
Greiner Bio-One Vacuette N.A.
4238 Capital Drive
Monroe, NC 28110

Rev 01. T040103

TABLE 2.2 ■ The Most Common Additives, Their Function, Use, and Limitations

Additive	Position in the Clinical and Laboratory Standards Institute Order of Draw*	Color of Stopper	Component Tested	Function of Additive	Tests Commonly Performed	Precautions (See Chapter 6)
Sodium citrate	2	Blue	Plasma	Binds or chelates calcium	Coagulation studies (PT, aPTT, factor assays)	Must fill to at least 90% of stated volume. Discard tube optional
Clot activator (e.g., silica)	3	Red	Serum	Promotes clotting	Chemistry, serology, immunology, blood bank**	Facilitates complete clotting, not faster clotting
Clot activator with gel	3	Red, gold, speckled	Serum	Promotes clotting (activator) and separates serum from cells (gel)	Chemistry, serology, immunology, blood bank,** TDMs**	Not recommended for progesterone or tricyclic antidepressants
Heparin (sodium, lithium, or ammonium)	4	Green	Plasma or whole blood	Inhibits thrombin activation by activating antithrombin III	Stat and routine chemistry	Avoid drawing lithium levels into lithium heparin tube
EDTA (K₂ or K₃)	5	Lavender, pink	Plasma or whole blood	Binds or chelates calcium	CBC, Blood Bank	Underfilling leads to excessive anticoagulation and erroneous results
Sodium fluoride, sodium, or potassium oxalate	6	Gray	Plasma	Precipitates calcium (sodium oxalate) and prevents glycolysis (sodium fluoride)	Glucose	Preserves glucose levels for at least 1 week
Sodium citrate	(not specified)	Black	Whole blood	Binds or chelates calcium	Sedimentation rate	

*Blood cultures are always collected first in the order of draw.

**Not all manufacturer's clot activator tubes are FDA cleared for this application. Refer to manufacturer for limitations.

volume less than 90% fill will falsely elevate aPTT results (1). Similarly, prothrombin times are inaccurate in therapeutic ranges if filled less than 80% and inaccurate on normal patients when filled less than 65%.

Immediate inversion of these specimens is critical to fully anticoagulate the specimen. Equally critical, blue stopper tubes must be drawn before any other tube with an additive to prevent carryover that could affect clotting studies. (See "Order of Draw," Chapter 3.)

 Tips from the Trenches: *Immediate inversion of sodium citrate tubes is critical to fully anticoagulate the specimen.*

Clot Activator (Serum) Tube

Glass activates the clotting mechanism (Fig. 2.2). When collection tubes are made of plastic, an additive is required to facilitate the clotting process so that serum can be obtained. Compounds that facilitate clotting include silica or glass particles with surface areas that activate the clotting mechanism. These clot activators don't necessarily hasten clotting, but facilitate full clotting rendering a fibrin-free specimen after centrifugation. As in glass tubes, full clotting can take up to 30 minutes. Clot activator tubes yield serum for a multitude of chemistry, serology, and immunology tests.

Some clot activator tubes also contain a thixotropic gel barrier to facilitate separation of the serum from the cells during centrifugation. As the force of centrifugation increases, the gel becomes liquid, migrates to the interface of the serum and cells, and resolidifies to provide a barrier that prevents contact. The thixotropic gels inserted in the tubes by most manufacturers are inert and impart no interference to test results. However, those of some manufacturers affect results when therapeutic drug monitoring (TDMs) is conducted on stored serum. Before drawing TDMs in gel tubes, refer to manufacturer's recommendations for limitations that may exist on gel tubes in use in your facility.

Serum from gel tubes is not to be used for testing progesterone DATs and tricyclic antidepressants (2).

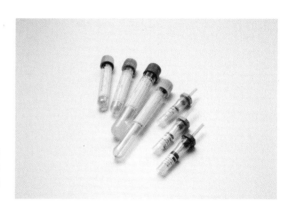

FIGURE 2.2 A wide variety of tube sizes should be available for draws that yield limited volumes of blood.

Heparin Tube—Green Stopper

Heparin prevents clotting by inhibiting thrombin activation, which is required in order for the coagulation cascade to unfold and produce a clot. Green stopper heparin tubes can contain sodium, lithium, or ammonium heparin. Heparinized tubes are considered a great convenience in stat situations where turnaround time is critical. Since heparinized specimens do not clot, specimens can be centrifuged immediately and the plasma tested, eliminating the delay necessitated for serum tubes to clot before centrifugation.

However, not as many routine tests can be performed on plasma as can be performed on serum. Collectors must not collect ammonia levels into ammonia heparin tubes or lithium blood levels into lithium heparin tubes. In both cases, the additive will significantly and falsely elevate test results. However, it is generally thought that sodium heparin does not impart a significant contribution to the sodium level reported on plasma from a sodium heparin tube. Some argue the level of sodium in the blood is of such a magnitude that the comparatively minute quantity in a sodium heparin tube does not increase the result to a significant degree. However, not all facilities accept this premise. Follow the protocol your facility has established when collecting electrolytes or other chemistry panels that include sodium into sodium heparin tubes. Some heparin tubes also contain a gel separator to facilitate separation of plasma from cells.

EDTA Tube—Lavender Stopper

No other anticoagulant preserves cellular integrity or prevents platelet aggregation as well as EDTA, making it the anticoagulant of choice for hematologic and immunologic tests. EDTA, or ethylenediaminetetraacetic acid, disrupts the clotting process by binding calcium, an essential element for clotting to occur. Tubes containing EDTA have a lavender or pink stopper, depending on their use.

Lavender stopper EDTA tubes contain powdered K_2 (di-potassium) or liquid K_3 (tri-potassium) salts and must be inverted 8 to 10 times upon filling. These tubes remain well mixed and are not centrifuged prior to testing. Most standards organizations recognize K_2 EDTA as the anticoagulant of choice for blood cell counts. Although not as sensitive to underfilling as sodium citrate tubes, underfilled EDTA tubes cause red blood cell (RBC) shrinkage due to excessive anticoagulation. As a result, the hematocrit, mean corpuscular volume (MCV), and red cell distribution width (RDW) will be falsely decreased, presenting an erroneous picture to the physician. Transporting significantly underfilled EDTA tubes to the testing facility for complete blood counts (CBCs) challenges testing personnel to uphold the facility's testing standards and risks a delay in reporting the results due to recollection when the specimen is ultimately rejected.

K_2 and K_3 EDTA with a pink stopper are used to perform immunohematologic (blood bank) testing and may be centrifuged to separate plasma for testing.

Sodium Fluoride/Oxalate Tube–Gray Stopper

Gray stopper sodium fluoride/oxalate tubes are ideal for preserving glucose levels in specimens drawn remote to the testing facility when transportation prevents immediate testing. Sodium oxalate removes calcium by precipitating it instead of binding or chelating it. Sodium fluoride preserves the glucose level by preventing glycolysis, the metabolism of glucose by the RBCs. This anticoagulant is also helpful in preserving blood alcohol levels. It is important to draw this tube as the last tube in the order of draw since carry-over of the anticoagulant can alter RBC morphology (lavender stopper), potassium (red, gold, speckled, or green stopper) and coagulation studies (blue stopper). (See "Order of Draw," Chapter 3.)

 Tips from the Trenches: Because the small bore of 25-gauge needles may hemolyze RBCs as they pass through, healthcare personnel should avoid their use for blood collection. The potential for hemolysis increases if a vacuum or excessive negative pressure is applied as during syringe use.

Needle Selection

Proper needle selection is critical to a successful venipuncture. A wide variety of sizes are available for venipuncture use, although some are limited to specific procedures. The largest, 16 to 18 gauge, are reserved for drawing large quantities of blood (e.g., blood donation or for use in therapeutic phlebotomy in which an entire unit of blood is drawn from a patient). Nineteen- to 20-gauge needles are used to minimize the activation of platelets during the collection of platelet aggregations studies, but are too large and painful for routine venipunctures. For routine specimen collection, 21- to 23-gauge needles are most commonly used. However, the bore of a 21-gauge needle is still relatively large. If patient comfort is of concern, preference should be given to a 22- or 23-gauge needle. These sizes are ideal for most punctures because it provides a good blood flow with little or no discomfort to the patient upon insertion when proper technique is used.

The 23-gauge needle is preferred for pediatric draws, hand veins, or veins that appear fragile or problematic. In addition, its size provides an extra measure of comfort. Draws with 23-gauge needles are less likely to result in the collapse of small, delicate veins or to traumatize the fragile veins of geriatric patients.

Healthcare personnel should avoid the use of 25-gauge needles for blood collection. Its small bore may result in the hemolysis of the RBCs as they pass through, especially if a vacuum or excessive syringe pressure is applied.

Syringes, Tube Holders, and Winged Collection Sets

One of the first decisions blood collectors have to make is whether to use a tube holder, a syringe, or a winged collection ("butterfly") set to collect the specimen. Each system has its benefits and drawbacks including safety, cost, and ease-of-use. The site selected for the puncture often dictates the equipment to be used.

Using a needle/syringe assembly allows the collector to control the pressure applied within veins that appear fragile or are of small diameter. Syringe use permits the collector to pull back on the plunger as slowly as necessary to maintain blood flow into the barrel of the syringe. Should the pressure of pulling the plunger become excessive during the collection and collapse the vein, the operator can reduce pulling pressure, which can release the occlusion and restore blood flow into the syringe. This ability to control the pressure is critical to successful punctures on smaller diameter veins and on veins outside the antecubital area.

However, if blood fills the barrel of the syringe too slowly because the needle is not completely within the vein, excessive pulling pressure on the plunger can hemolyze RBCs, rendering the specimen unacceptable. Likewise, a specimen collected too slowly can begin to clot in the barrel of the syringe. This condition not only makes it difficult to evacuate the specimen into the collection tubes when the puncture is complete, but can also introduce microclots into the specimen, which cause erroneous results when undetected by testing personnel.

A final benefit of using a syringe is the visible "flash" of blood into the hub of the syringe indicating the vein has been accessed. Healthcare professionals should be cautioned not to rely on this flash exclusively as an indication of a successful puncture, however, because the absence of a flash of blood into the hub does not necessarily indicate the needle is not in place. Low blood pressure, a loose tourniquet, and other factors can prevent a visible flash of blood into the syringe from occurring when the needle is within the vein. Therefore, a visible flash of blood is not a completely reliable indicator of venous access, and healthcare personnel should be cautioned against relying on this feature as proof of venous access.

 According to the Standards . . . draws using syringes should be avoided due to the high frequency of accidental needlesticks associated with syringe use.

The most common method of drawing blood on prominent veins of the antecubital area is with the use of a tube holder (Fig. 2.3). This device allows the vacuum of the tube to withdraw the specimen from the vein quickly and effortlessly. The convenience and ease of use of this system appeal to many healthcare personnel with specimen collection responsibilities. However, vacuum-assisted draws are not appropriate for use on all veins of all patients. Although the benefits of tube holders are undisputed on prominent veins in the antecubital area where most venipunctures take place, they have limited usefulness on smaller veins in other areas.

Unlike syringe draws, the use of tube holders does not allow collectors to control the vacuum applied to the inside of the vein. When the tube is applied, the full force of the vacuum within the tube is transferred to the interior of the vein. Even though the vacuum decreases proportionately as the

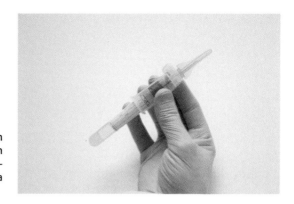

FIGURE 2.3 The most common method of drawing blood on prominent veins of the antecubital area is with the use of a tube holder.

tube fills, the initial force of the vacuum to the inside of the vein can cause the vein to collapse. This occurs in veins lacking patency (common in geriatric patients) and when the space between the beveled opening of the needle and the inner wall of the vein is minimal. When the vacuum of the tube is transferred to the interior of the vein, the wall of the vein can be pulled onto the beveled opening of the needle occluding it and preventing blood from filling the tube. Therefore, tube holder assemblies should only be used on the large-diameter veins of the antecubital area or on smaller veins only when smaller volume tubes are available. Understanding the limitations of the equipment when selecting the puncture site is critical to a successful venipuncture.

 Tips from the Trenches: Veins collapse when collectors select a needle-tube combination that is inappropriate for the size and patency of the vein.

Winged blood collection sets, also known as "butterfly" sets, are preferred by many healthcare professionals as blood collection devices. Their lightweight design makes them easy to manipulate, and their wings allow a lower angle of insertion and greater control than what a syringe or tube holder can offer. Like syringes, winged collection sets allow the operator to see an immediate flash of blood in the tubing, indicating that the vein has been successfully accessed. However, the absence of this flash does not mean that the vein has not been accessed.

However convenient, winged collection sets have significant drawbacks as routine devices for blood collection. In some winged collection sets, the cut of the bevel is much more blunt than that of standard needles and can result in a more painful puncture. In addition, winged collection sets are considerably more expensive to use than conventional devices, are too short to reach deep veins, and are associated with an inordinately high rate of accidental needlesticks. One study (conducted before OSHA mandated safety needles) showed that winged collection sets were responsible for 35% of all accidental needlesticks to phlebotomists (3). Although winged collection sets now have a safety feature designed to protect the healthcare worker, their effectiveness depends on user activation. Because of these limitations, healthcare professionals should use these devices only when special circumstances make them necessary, such as when attempting to access fragile or small veins of geriatric and pediatric patients.

EQUIPMENT ASSEMBLY

Tube Holders

Before assembling needles and tube holders, inspect the paper seal of the needle, which manufacturers apply to assure their sterility. If the seal is broken, its sterility is in question and the needle must be discarded. To prepare the needle for assembly, hold the needle at opposite ends and twist the smaller protective cap off exposing a tight-fitting vinyl sleeve that encases the short "back end" of the needle. Discard the cap. Thread the exposed end into the threads of the tube holder. If the needle is exposed and comes in contact with any surface at any point during the assembly, its sterility is lost and the needle must be discarded.

Syringes

If choosing a syringe for the venipuncture, ensure the sterility of the device. This can be accomplished two ways:

1. Inspect the outer wrapper or casing to assure it has not been opened. If the syringe is packaged in a protective hard plastic casing, you should hear an audible click when opening the casing (Fig. 2.4).
2. Make sure the plunger seal is not broken. Plungers on unused syringes offer some resistance when used for the first time. Push or pull on the plunger to unseat it. Initial resistance followed by a freeing from the seal ensures the sterility of the device as long as the packaging is intact as described previously. If plunger resistance cannot be detected, discard the syringe and inspect another.

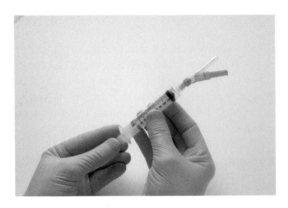

FIGURE 2.4 Break the seal of the syringe by pulling back to unseat the plunger, and then expel all the air by advancing it fully forward.

Remove the appropriate needle from its packaging. (See "Needle Selection," later in this chapter.) If the packaging is not intact or the seal is broken, the sterility of the needle cannot be guaranteed and the needle should be discarded. Remove the protective caps from the hub of the syringe (if present) and luer end of the needle. Attach the needle onto the syringe leaving the protective sheath in place until ready to perform the puncture.

Winged Collection Sets

Winged collection sets must always be used in conjunction with a syringe or tube holder. If the packaging of the set has been previously opened, discard it and use an unopened set. To attach a syringe, first ensure the sterility of the syringe as indicated previously, then assemble it onto the luer end of the winged collection set. Remove the adapter prior to attaching a syringe (Fig. 2.5, top). Unseat the plunger of the syringe and advance it fully forward, expelling the air from the barrel of the syringe.

To attach a tube holder, thread or attach the back end of the winged collection set to the tube holder (Fig. 2.5, bottom). (Some winged collection sets are prepackaged with adapters for threading onto tube holders.)

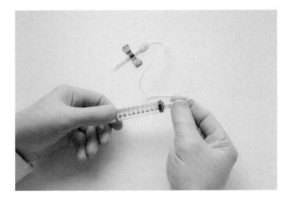

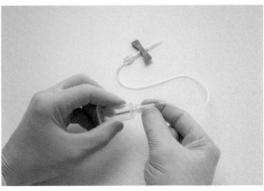

FIGURE 2.5 Attach either a syringe (top) or tube (bottom) holder to the back end of the winged collection set.

REFERENCES

1. Reneke J, Etzell J, Leslie S, et al. Prolonged prothrombin time and activated partial thromboplastin time due to underfilled specimen tubes with 109 mmol/L (3.2%) citrate anticoagulant. *Am J Clin Pathol* 1998;109:754–757.
2. NCCLS. *Procedures for the handling and processing of blood specimens.* Approved Standard, H18-A3, Wayne, PA, 2004.
3. Jagger J. Risky procedure, risky devices, risky job. *Adv Exposure Prev* 1994;1:4–9.

REVIEW QUESTIONS

1. Hemolysis refers to:
   a. the rupture of RBCs resulting in the tingeing of the serum or plasma with the hemoglobin pigment
   b. the pooling of blood beneath the surface of the skin
   c. the concentration of cells and larger molecules in the blood stream when the tourniquet is left on longer than 1 minute
   d. blood in the interstitial spaces
2. If supplies or equipment, such as tourniquets or gauze, fall to the floor in patient view:
   a. pick it up and use it on the patient
   b. leave it on the floor for housekeeping to discard
   c. pick it up and return it to your tray for later use
   d. dispose of the material in front of the patient
3. The 23-gauge needle is preferred for:
   a. draws to the median cubital vein
   b. platelet aggregation studies
   c. pediatric draws, hand veins, or veins that appear fragile or problematic
   d. obese patients
4. Disadvantages of winged blood collection sets include:
   a. a cut that is more blunt than that of standard needles
   b. are significantly more expensive
   c. associated with an inordinately high rate of accidental needlesticks
   d. all of the above
5. Tubes that contain a gel serum separator should not be used for:
   a. cholesterol testing
   b. progesterone testing
   c. pediatric patients
   d. VDRL testing
6. Most standards organizations recognize _____ as the anticoagulant of choice for blood cell counts.
   a. sodium citrate
   b. sodium fluoride
   c. K_2 EDTA
   d. K_3 EDTA
7. Plasma is:
   a. the liquid portion of the blood after centrifugation of a specimen that is allowed to clot
   b. the liquid portion of the blood after centrifugation of a specimen that has been anticoagulated
   c. blood that is well mixed with its cellular components
   d. the liquid portion of the blood that is used for cell counts

8. Heparin tubes are identified by their:
   a. red stopper
   b. green stopper
   c. blue stopper
   d. yellow/gold stopper
9. When red-stopper collection tubes are made of plastic, an additive is required to:
   a. prevent clotting
   b. prevent plastic polymers from leeching into the specimen
   c. bind calcium
   d. facilitate clotting

Performing the Venipuncture 3

KEY TERMS AND DEFINITIONS

Fasting 10- to 12-hour overnight dietary restriction of all intake except water and medications.

Hematoma The pooling of blood beneath the skin from ruptured veins, arteries, or capillaries. Identified by a raising or mounding of the tissue with or without immediate discoloration.

Hemoconcentration The static pooling of blood within the veins below venous constriction due to prolonged tourniquet application. During hemoconcentration, large molecules (e.g., proteins), coagulation factors, and cells accumulate disproportionately. Specimens drawn from hemoconcentrated veins may not reflect the patient's actual status. Hemoconcentration begins affecting test results within 1 minute of tourniquet application.

Vein palpation Lightly pressing down on the skin repeatedly with varying degrees of pressure to detect underlying veins. Too much pressure may not allow for the tactile sensation of the vein's curvature or elasticity. Likewise, too little pressure may not bring the finger close enough to feel the vein.

Note: This section assumes a puncture in the antecubital area. Because technique is site-specific, refer to "Alternative Sites" in Chapter 4 for variations in the basic technique specific for draws outside of the antecubital area.

INTRODUCTION

Those who collect blood specimens for clinical testing have a responsibility to the patient that goes beyond simply obtaining a blood sample. Adhering to the acceptable standards for venipuncture is critical in obtaining specimens free from errors that can affect results and protecting patients from injury. Healthcare personnel are cautioned to comply with the established standards and their facility's procedure in order to be protected from the liability of performing beneath the standard of care.

This chapter details the routine venipuncture using a syringe, tube holder, and winged collection set. The type of device used depends on a multitude of variables discussed in Chapter 2. After reading this chapter, the reader should be able to:

- List the steps of a properly performed venipuncture
- State the acceptable means of patient identification according to Clinical and Laboratory Standards Institute (formerly NCCLS)
- Identify safe practices when performing a routine venipuncture
- State the importance of minimizing preanalytical errors during specimen collection
- State the proper order in which tubes should be filled
- Discuss the effects that underfilling collection tubes has on test results
- Describe the limitations of needle manipulation when the vein is not initially accessed
- Identify the vein of the antecubital that lies in closest proximity to the nerve most often injured during venipunctures
- Select a vein of the antecubital area that reduces the risk of injury to the patient to its lowest possible degree

SAFETY

Collectors should carefully select the equipment that is most suitable for the draw based on the patient's condition and vein accessibility. Proper personal protective equipment (PPE) is essential to protect the healthcare professional from injury and exposure. According to OSHA, gloves must be worn whenever drawing blood for clinical testing without exception. (See Box 3.1, "OSHA Standard Precautions," and Box 3.2, "Glove Use.") Eye protection and impermeable gowns or clothing must be worn whenever the employer determines that exposure to blood or other potentially infectious material (OPIM) is possible. Failure to use recommended PPEs subjects the employee to an increased risk of exposure and the employer to OSHA citations and fines.

In the interest of the inpatient's well-being, avoid placing the phlebotomy tray on patient care surfaces such as the bedside tray. The underside of phlebotomy trays may carry a host of bacteria that can be transferred to surfaces patients use frequently. (See "Bug Bombs" in the Phlebotomy Tip of the Month section of the Appendices.)

BOX 3.1 ▪ Standard Precautions

According to OSHA, "Universal precautions shall be observed to prevent contact with blood or other potentially infectious materials"(10). Defined by the Centers for Disease Control and Prevention (CDC) and OSHA, "Universal Precautions" (now referred to as "standard precautions") refers to a method of infection control in which all human blood and certain body fluids are treated as if known to be infectious for HIV, HBV, and other bloodborne pathogens. Practices that reflect Standard Precautions include (1):

- Washing hands before and after patient care or if bodily fluids have been handled
- Wearing gloves whenever contact with body substances, mucous membranes, or nonintact skin is possible
- Wearing gowns impermeable to liquids when clothing is likely to become soiled or contaminated with body fluids
- Wearing a mask and protective eyewear or a face shield when the risk of being splashed with body fluids exists
- Placing intact needles, syringe units, and/or sharps in a designated disposal container as soon as possible without recapping
- Not breaking or bending needles
- Refraining from all direct patient care and the handling of patient care equipment if you have a weeping rash. (See "Having a Pathogen Pitch-In?" and "Taking Work Home With You" in the Phlebotomy Tip of the Month section of the Appendices.)

BOX 3.2 ▪ Glove Use: It's Not Just for Your Safety

According to OSHA, gloves must be worn whenever drawing blood for clinical testing without exception. However, OSHA does not specify when gloves must be put on. Some facilities allow gloveless palpation providing the patient is not in isolation and the individual exercises proper hand hygiene between patients. However, gloves must always be worn when the vein is accessed.

Although gloves do not prevent an accidental needlestick, they can prevent an exposure should the patient bleed unexpectedly. Consider the following hypothetical situation: you are drawing blood without gloves. The needle is within the vein and the blood is filling the tubes. Suddenly, the patient jerks unexpectedly, or someone enters the room and bumps you from behind. The needle comes out of the vein and blood pools on the skin. Instinctively, you loosen the tourniquet, reach for the gauze, and apply pressure to the puncture site. Enough blood had pooled on the skin to saturate the gauze through to your bare fingers. Just like everyone else, the skin of your fingers has breaks from paper cuts, chapping, scrapes, etc. that occur from routine use. The breaks in your skin provide a port for hepatitis, HIV, or other organisms to enter your system.

Unless you can guarantee that every venipuncture you perform will be routine and without incident, drawing blood without gloves risks not only your life, but the lives of all those who love you and depend upon you.

PREANALYTICAL ERRORS

It has been estimated that physicians receive 70% of the objective information on their patients' health status from laboratory results (2). Therefore, it is critical that test results are not altered by improper specimen collection. Those who collect specimens can significantly affect test results and cause patients to be misdiagnosed, over- or undermedicated, or otherwise mismanaged. The effect can be life-threatening. Up to 56% of all errors that can affect a blood specimen or the test result occur during the collection and processing phase (3). Such "preanalytical" errors cost the average 400-bed hospital $200,000 per year in re-collections and medication errors (4).

Table 3.1 summarizes the types of errors that occur most often, have the greatest impact on patient management, and are easiest for healthcare personnel to control. Those who are aware of them and work to prevent them can keep the impact of these errors on patient results to a minimum. Applying the principles of specimen collection, processing, and transport, as reflected in the Clinical and Laboratory Standards Institute standards and throughout this book, is critical to assure physicians that the information they receive on their patients' status is accurate.

PATIENT IDENTIFICATION

Properly identifying patients is the most important step in specimen collection (Box 3.3). When standard procedures for patient identification are compromised or a patient's identity is assumed, specimen collection personnel can be responsible for patient overmedication, undermedication, general mismanagement, or even death (Fig. 3.1).

TABLE 3.1 ▪ Preanalytical Errors

Before Collection	During Collection	After Collection
Patient misidentification	Prolonged tourniquet time	Failure to separate serum from cells
Improper time of collection	Hemolysis	Improper use of serum separators
Wrong tube	Order of draw	Processing delays
Inadequate fast	Failure to invert tubes	Exposure to light
Exercise	Faulty technique	Improper storage conditions
Patient posture	Underfilling tubes	Rimming clots
Poor coordination with other treatments		
Nonsterile site preparation		
Not coordinating with medication		

BOX 3.3   Identifying Patients

When identifying patients, do not:

- Assume the information on the identification bracelet is correct
- Assume the patient is in the room or bed indicated on the requisition
- Ask patients to affirm their name as in "Are you John Smith?"
- Rely on bed tags, crib cards, water pitchers, charts, or identification bracelets that are not attached to the patient
- Assume the outpatient that responds to the name you call out is actually the intended patient
- Draw a patient without an arm bracelet until the appropriate caregiver has provided the patient's name, address, date of birth, and/or unique identification number
- Assume the unconscious patient is the intended patient without verification from the appropriate caregiver or family member

It Could Happen to You

Two patients were admitted into the same room at the same time. The admitting nurse mistakenly switched their arm bracelets so that the patient in bed A was identified as the patient in bed B and vice versa. Twenty-four hours later, a laboratory technologist entered the room to draw peak vancomycin levels on each patient. The identification bracelet of the patient in bed A matched the requisition. However, when asked to state his name, the name given didn't match and the error was finally discovered.

Question: How did the collector prevent a mistake that could have resulted in a medication error?

Answer: Because the technologist asked the patient to state his name, the identification bracelet error was discovered. Had he not followed the standard protocol for patient identification and relied solely on the arm bracelet, each patient would likely have been treated according to the other's vancomycin level.

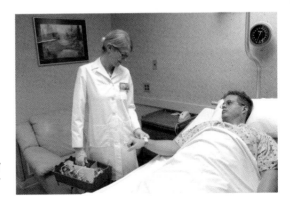

FIGURE 3.1 Failing to properly identify patients is a potentially fatal specimen collection error.

Inpatient Identification

It is of paramount importance for the healthcare professional to ensure that the specimen drawn is from the intended patient. However, relying on arm bracelets alone is not sufficient. One study showed that up to 16% of arm bracelets have erroneous information (4). To avoid inpatient misidentification, the Clinical and Laboratory Standards Institute recommends (5):

1. Asking the patient to state his/her full name, address, birth date, and/or unique identification number.
2. Comparing the information given with the information on the patient's identification bracelet (which must be attached to the patient) and the test requisition.
3. Reporting any discrepancy to the appropriate caregiver according to facility policy and having the caregiver identify the patient by name and identification number before drawing the specimen.

 According to the Standards . . . discrepancies in patient identification must be reported to the responsible caregiver who must identify the patient by name and identification number before the specimen is drawn.

Under no circumstances should the patient's identity be assumed on the basis of his/her location. For example, a requisition shows the patient John Williams to be in Bed 1. If the patient in Bed 1 is incoherent or unresponsive and does not have an identifying bracelet affixed to him, it is dangerous to assume that John Williams is indeed the patient in Bed 1.

If a patient's identification bracelet is not affixed to their person (i.e., wrist or ankle), the bracelet cannot be considered a reliable source of identification. Likewise, patient names written on water pitchers, bed tags, or posted charts do not constitute valid patient identification (Fig. 3.2). Should an arm bracelet be found attached to the bedrail, foot of the bed, or on the bedside

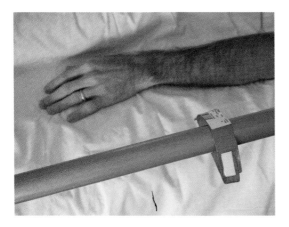

FIGURE 3.2 Unless attached to the patient, arm bracelets must not be considered as a reliable form of identification. (From the Center for Phlebotomy Education, with permission.)

table, the patient's caregiver should be notified and reapply the bracelet to the patient prior to drawing the specimen. If the identification bracelet is not available or if conditions exist that preclude the application of an identification bracelet (e.g., severely burned patients, residents in long-term care facilities, etc.), the patient's immediate caregiver must provide positive patient identification in the form of the patient's name, address, birth date, and/or unique identification number. Document the name of the verifier in case the patient is misidentified.

 Tips from the Trenches: *Those who draw blood from long-term care facility residents who do not have identification bracelets must obtain verification of patient identification from the resident's immediate caregiver and document the name of the verifier.*

If the patient is unconscious, without language skills (e.g., infants), cognitively impaired, or does not speak the language of the collector, the nurse or a relative/friend should identify the patient by name, address, date of birth, and/or unique identification number. The information provided should be compared with that on the requisition and, in the case of inpatients, with the patient's attached identification bracelet. Any discrepancies must be resolved by the appropriate caregiver before the specimen is collected.

Healthcare personnel responsible for collecting specimens from newborns and infants must be especially careful not to rely on crib cards for identification. As with adults without Bracelets, the infant's caregiver must provide positive identification and the name of the verifier should be documented.

When asking patients to state their name, avoid the temptation to ask them to affirm the name you provide as in "Are you Mr. Smith?" Patients who have difficulty hearing or who may have altered mental states due to medication or other conditions may respond in the affirmative without understanding the question.

 According to the Standards *. . . inpatient identification consists of comparing the information on the patient's identification bracelet with the requisitions and asking the patient to state his/her name, address, identification number, and/or date of birth.*

When drawing blood from unidentified emergency patients when the patient's condition does not allow a delay in specimen collection, a unique temporary identifier in the form of a number or other designation should be assigned to the patient until proper identification has been established and is in place. The temporary identifier should be included on all requisitions and specimens. When a permanent identification number has been assigned, the temporary number should be cross-referenced in a timely manner to the permanent number such that the patient's results are accurately attributed without compromising patient care.

Outpatient Identification

Healthcare professionals should not rely completely on the papers that an outpatient brings to the drawing station for identification. For outpatients, the Clinical and Laboratory Standards Institute states:

- Ask the patient to state his/her full name, address, date of birth, and/or unique identification number.
- Compare the information given with the information on the request form.
- Report any discrepancy to the appropriate caregiver according to facility policy and have him/her identify the patient by name and identification number before drawing the specimen.

Resist the temptation to consider a patient's response to the name you call out in the waiting area as confirmation of his name. As with inpatients, similar sounding names can be confused and affirmation of the name called out does not constitute proper patient identification.

Outpatients who have come in for possible transfusions should be identified with a unique arm bracelet that establishes and maintains their identification for possible transfusion at a later time.

Adhere to the Clinical and Laboratory Standards Institute standards and facility policy when identifying all patients. Failure to follow the established protocol for patient identification can result in medical errors and patient death.

CONFIRM TEST REQUIREMENTS

If the requested test(s) require certain patient conditions to be met (e.g., fasting, time of medication administration, patient to be recumbent, etc.), confirm the requirements are met. For example, if the patient is being drawn for a fasting test such as a fasting glucose or lipid profile, ask the patient if he/she has had anything to eat that day. If the patient does not meet the conditions required by the test or the physician's orders, reschedule the test or consult with the physician or the patient's immediate caregiver. Document the patient's conditions pertinent to the test to provide the physician with the information necessary to interpret the test(s) properly.

POSITION THE PATIENT

Outpatient

Typically, outpatients are seated in specially designed phlebotomy chairs at permanent drawing stations (Fig. 3.3). According to the Clinical and Laboratory Standards Institute, venipunctures should be performed in a clean, quiet, private environment. Phlebotomy chairs that provide maximum security and comfort for both phlebotomist and patient are recommended. Ergonomically designed chairs are available that adjust vertically, bringing patients to the

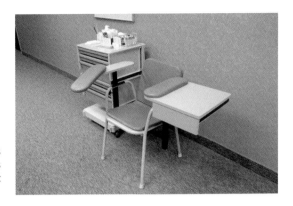

FIGURE 3.3 Phlebotomy chairs should have adjustable armrests to provide support and prevent falls.

optimum working height for the collector. This feature prevents back injuries that are the result of repeatedly bending down too far to work at a comfortable distance. Adjustable armrests are necessary to provide support and prevent patients who lose consciousness from falling. If the patient expresses a tendency to faint during blood collection procedures, a bed should be available nearby and the patient allowed to lay down during the procedure.

When drawing specimens in a patient's home, make sure the patient's arm is supported on a solid surface and that the chair in which the patient is seated has armrests should the patient lose consciousness. If a chair with armrests is not available, have the patient recline on a sofa or bed. Request that patients remove gum, food, and foreign objects from the mouth during the procedure.

 According to the Standards . . . venipunctures should be performed in a clean, quiet, private environment with a phlebotomy chair that provides maximum security and comfort for both phlebotomist and patient including adjustable armrests to prevent fainting patients from falling.

Inpatient

Inpatients who are not recumbent on a bed or gurney should be seated in a chair with armrests. Avoid drawing blood from patients seated on the bed. Should the patient lose consciousness during or after the draw, a fall could result in serious injury. All patients should be asked to remove gum, food and foreign objects from the mouth during the puncture.

VENIPUNCTURE PROCEDURE

Site Selection

The most common site for performing a venipuncture is the antecubital area of the arm (*ante* comes from the Latin word for "before"; *cubital* from the Latin for "elbow") because of the accessibility of several large veins: the medial (consisting of the median, median cephalic, and median cubital veins), the cephalic, and the basilic. These veins pass through this area in a generally predictable course and are usually visible or palpable. However, many factors must be taken into consideration before selecting the antecubital area as the site for a venipuncture.

Necessity for Restraint

Patients who are cognitively or emotionally impaired may require restraint prior to performing a venipuncture. If restraint is necessary, the arm may be difficult to immobilize because of the joint at the antecubital area. In extremely combative or resistant patients it may be prudent to draw from an alternative site. (Because patients have the right to refuse procedures including venipunctures, refer to Chapter 2, Patient Bill of Rights, before drawing specimens from a combative or resistant patient.)

Mastectomy Patients

If the patient had a mastectomy, punctures in the arm on the same side are not permitted without physician approval (5). Significant lymph node removal often accompanies surgical mastectomy procedures. Because lymph nodes regulate fluid balance, their removal effectively interferes with lymph flow (lymphostasis) in the respective limb. In addition, blood collected from the same side as a mastectomy may contain higher concentrations of lymphocytes and waste products normally contained in the lymph fluid (6).

More importantly to the patient, any infection in the affected limb can result in excruciating pain from edema, which can last for months. Patients who have undergone mastectomies, therefore, can have significant and painful consequences from even the most minor infections and must be protected from even the smallest breaks in the skin. Most mastectomy patients will be acutely aware of the potential complications and will inform the phlebotomist before a puncture is attempted. These circumstances should be taken seriously.

Availability of Veins

Most patients have six potentially acceptable veins in their combined antecubital areas. In some patients, though, it can be difficult to locate even one. Age, obesity, dehydration, chemotherapy, and many other medical conditions and treatments can be factors that make finding antecubital veins difficult.

Collector's Skill

Not all healthcare personnel have the confidence to puncture veins they can feel but can't see. Those new to the procedure or those who perform venipunctures infrequently often consider alternative sites. However, as one's phlebotomy skills improve and one becomes more reliant on the sense of touch than sight, confidence in performing antecubital venipunctures increases.

Presence of Edema

Because swelling makes locating veins more difficult and can prolong healing and closure of the puncture site, venipunctures should be avoided in an arm with edema. Additionally, excessive swelling can alter the composition of the blood collected from the affected limb.

Injuries

Venipunctures to an arm that is injured, burned, scarred, or otherwise traumatized should be avoided. Nor should infected, inflamed, or excessively bruised antecubital areas be considered. Patients who had a stroke may have a limited ability to hyperextend the arm, thereby preventing access to the antecubital area.

Infusion of Intravenous Fluids

Since intravenous fluid infusion threatens to contaminate specimens, draws from the same arm as fluids are being infused should be avoided. (See "Venipunctures and IV Infusions," Chapter 4.)

If any of these conditions preclude the use of the antecubital area, an alternative site should be considered. (See Chapter 4.)

 Tips from the Trenches: Because even the most minor infections can bring significant and painful consequences to patients who have undergone mastectomies, they must be protected from even the smallest breaks in the skin.

It Could Happen to You

A physician ordered intravenous (IV) therapy for an inpatient who had undergone a prior mastectomy. She informed the nurse of her condition, but the nurse inserted the cannula into the affected arm nonetheless. The patient experienced a fluid imbalance in the limb resulting in excruciating pain and discomfort for months. She sued the facility employing the nurse for violations against the standard of care.

Question: How could this injury have been prevented?

Answer: By avoiding invasive procedures to the arm affected by a prior mastectomy, healthcare personnel prevent the painful lymphedema that can occur. Punctures (venipunctures and fingersticks) to the same side as a prior mastectomy should never be performed without the written permission of the patient's physician.

VEIN SELECTION

Begin by tightening a tourniquet several inches above the antecubital area. To assure patient comfort, it should not roll into a ropelike constrictor, but remain flat around the circumference of the upper arm. To avoid pinching the patient's skin, tighten the tourniquet around the patient's sleeve if possible. Tourniquets should be tight but not uncomfortable to the patient. Tuck a loop of the tourniquet between the tourniquet and the arm to provide an easy, one-handed release.

Latex tourniquets should be avoided to prevent allergic reactions and the development of latex sensitivities. Several other types of tourniquets currently are available including vinyl, nitrile, and cloth or rubber tourniquets with Velcro-type fasteners. Alternatively, a blood pressure cuff can be used in place of a tourniquet if inflated to a level below the patient's diastolic pressure (5). If the blood pressure is not known or cannot be taken, inflating the cuff to 40 mm Hg usually is adequate.

After applying constriction, instruct the patient to clench the fist. Discourage pumping of the fist as such activity can elevate levels of potassium and ionized calcium in the bloodstream (5). Pumping the fist also brings about movement in the antecubital area that can interfere with vein location.

Locate the most prominent of the three acceptable veins of the antecubital area visually and by palpation. The median, median cubital, and median cephalic veins (collectively known as "medial veins") typically lie in the center of the antecubital area; the cephalic vein is on the outside (lateral) aspect; the basilic is on the inside (medial) aspect of the antecubital area (Fig. 3.4). Palpate for each vein by pushing lightly on the skin with increasing pressure using the index finger. Veins will feel spongy, resilient, and have a tubelike curvature. Tendons and bone are harder structures and distinctively different. Attempt to locate a medial vein first. They are the veins of choice for several reasons:

1. Proximity—medial veins are typically the closest to the skin's surface, making them readily accessible.
2. Immobility—medial veins are also the most stationary of the antecubital veins and least likely to move when the needle is inserted making a successful puncture more probable.
3. Safety—punctures to the medial veins pose the least risk of injuring underlying structures.
4. Comfort—the medial veins bring less discomfort when punctured.

However, medial veins are only the veins of choice if they are visible or palpable and if there is a high degree of confidence they can be accessed successfully. Choosing another vein when a medial is clearly present can increase the patient's risk for injury. However, selecting an indistinct medial vein over one of the other clearly visible or palpable veins may result in an unsuccessful attempt and subject the patient to a second puncture unnecessarily.

If a medial vein cannot be located, palpate on the lateral (outer) aspect of the arm where the cephalic vein lies. Complete the survey by palpating the

BOX 3.4 ▦ Tourniquet Hygiene

Many facilities discard tourniquets after one use. Although not required by any regulatory agency, it's a good infection control practice and good customer service. Patients notice the cleanliness of supplies and equipment. Applying a dull, soiled, or blood-flecked tourniquet is disturbing to patients, whether they mention it or not. Take these steps to instill confidence in your patients that you have a healthy respect for their well-being:

■ If you drop a tourniquet on the floor, discard it. Picking up and using dropped supplies and equipment on your patients destroys their confidence in your contribution to their healing process. It tells them that you are unsanitary and without regard for their well-being. Probably none of these things are true, but that is the message it sends.

■ Discarding tourniquets contaminated with blood protects your patients from disease and from developing a bad impression of your facility. If a tourniquet is flecked with blood, discard it.

■ Nosocomial infections kill 75,000 patients every year (11). If you're not discarding tourniquets after every use, discard them after several uses or at least daily. Nosocomial infections, those spread from patient to patient by hospital staff, are the bane of every healthcare facility. Too often we think that proper hand washing is the only way to combat spreading infection. But discarding tourniquets after several uses is highly effective and helps give your patients a fighting chance to avoid a hospital-acquired infection.

■ If you wouldn't put it around the arm of your child, don't put it around the arm of a patient.

■ Think of tourniquets as disposable. . . because they are. (See "Tourniquet Hygiene" in the Phlebotomy Tip of the Month section of the Appendices.)

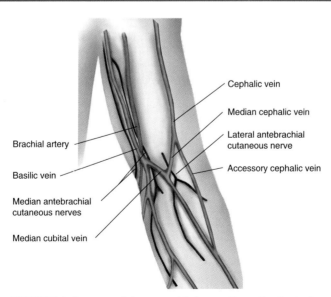

FIGURE 3.4 Anatomy of the antecubital area. (From the Center for Phlebotomy Education, with permission.)

skin on the medial (inner) aspect of the antecubital area where the basilic vein lies. Even if a cephalic or basilic vein has been located, repeat the survey on the opposite arm (if accessible) in an attempt to locate a medial vein. Healthcare personnel who select a basilic vein before surveying for a medial or cephalic vein do not reduce the risk of injury to the lowest possible degree (see Chapter 7). That's because two branches of an antebrachial cutaneous nerve lie in close proximity to the basilic vein, sometimes passing between the skin and the vein itself (7). Once pierced, these nerves send shooting pain down the length of the limb to the fingers, sometimes up to the shoulder and into the chest. Nerve injury is often disabling and can be permanent. Most nerve injuries that result from punctures in the antecubital area occur during attempts to puncture the basilic vein. Since nerves are neither visible nor palpable, avoiding the basilic vein when other prominent veins are available reduces the risk of nerve injury. (See "Of All the Nerve" in the Phlebotomy Tip of the Month section of the Appendices.)

 According to the Standards . . . "Attempt to locate a medial vein on either arm before considering alternative veins. Due to the proximity of the basilic vein to the brachial artery and the median nerve, this vein should only be considered if no other vein is more prominent."*

It Could Happen to You

After performing a thorough survey, a phlebotomist was presented with the option of puncturing a medial vein or the basilic vein. She chose the basilic vein and, because of poor technique, subsequently pierced a nerve that resulted in permanent injury to the patient. Partly because the phlebotomist chose the basilic vein when a medial vein was a well-defined option, the jury found the phlebotomist in error and awarded nearly $50,000 to the patient.

Question: How could this injury have been prevented?

Answer: Selecting a medial vein instead of the higher risk basilic vein would have reduced the risk of injury to the lowest possible degree. Although it is acceptable to puncture any of the three veins in the antecubital area, punctures to the basilic vein bring the greatest risk of injury due to its close proximity to nerves should the collector have poor technique or resort to probing.

*Reproduced with permission, from CLSI/NCCLS publication H3-A5-Procedures for the Collection of Diagnostic Blood Specimens by Venipuncture; Approved Standard-Fifth Edition (ISBN 1-56238-515-1). Copies of the current edition may be obtained from the Clinical and Laboratory Standards Institute, 940 West Valley Road, Suite 1400, Wayne, Pennsylvania 19087-1898, USA.

Tips from the Trenches: Always survey both arms with a tourniquet for the presence of the median or cephalic veins before choosing the higher risk basilic vein. Most nerve injuries that result from punctures in the antecubital area occur during attempts to puncture the basilic vein.

In addition to nerves, the basilic vein's close proximity to the brachial artery subjects the patient to the risk of an arterial nick and subsequent hemorrhage. Should this artery be pierced unknowingly, the consequences to the patient can range from a barely perceptible bruising to a severe hemorrhage, which if undetected, can lead to a compression nerve injury and other complications.

Nerves are delicate structures that can be damaged by the pressure that a hematoma exerts. When the pressure is significant and lasting, permanent injury can result. The most common diagnosis as a result of nerve compression is reflex sympathetic dystrophy, a painful condition that limits the use of the arm. Therefore, when considering punctures to the inside aspect of the antecubital area, collectors should attempt to locate the brachial artery by feeling for a pulse and avoid punctures in the area if the artery lies precariously close to the basilic vein.

When performing the survey for available veins in the antecubital area, it is common for only one or two veins to be located. Often the basilic is the patient's most prominent vein. Healthcare personnel must be aware, however, of the risk in accessing this vein and use it only when no other vein in the antecubital area is more accessible. Select the vein that offers the highest degree of confidence that it can be accessed safely and successfully, taking into consideration the risks involved.

Although those new to phlebotomy may only feel confident puncturing veins that are visible, this is a luxury not all patients provide. With time and repetition, confidence in attempting to access veins that are only palpable will increase. However, collectors should never blindly stick for a vein that is neither visible nor palpable.

It Could Happen to You

An outpatient came into the laboratory drawing station and was seated. The phlebotomist noticed a prominent basilic vein and punctured it without applying a tourniquet or even surveying either arm for the presence of a median or cephalic vein. The patient felt an excruciating, shooting pain upon needle insertion. He suffered permanent nerve damage and sued the facility for operating beneath the standard of care.

Question: How could this injury have been avoided?

Answer: By performing a thorough survey of both arms for the presence of a medial or cephalic vein using a tourniquet, healthcare personnel may find several prominent veins and make a choice based on the degree of risk associated with each option. Only then can the risk of injury be reduced to its lowest possible level.

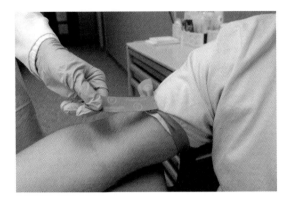

FIGURE 3.5 If vein selection alone takes longer than 1 minute, release the tourniquet and allow 2 minutes to pass before retightening it and performing the puncture.

 Tips from the Trenches: *"Blind sticking," that is, inserting a needle where veins are neither visible nor palpable, should never be attempted.*

Once a suitable vein has been selected, loosen the tourniquet and assemble the equipment (see Chapter 2). Leaving the tourniquet on longer than 1 minute causes hemoconcentration and alters the specimen before it is even collected (3,5,8–10). On patients with prominent veins, it may not be necessary to release the tourniquet as long as vein selection, equipment assembly, site cleansing, and venous access can be accomplished within 1 minute of tourniquet application. However, if it is anticipated that the process may take longer than 1 minute, release the tourniquet to prevent hemoconcentration and allow 2 minutes to pass before retightening it and performing the puncture (Fig. 3.5). This allows hemoconcentration to dissipate so that the specimen collected is an accurate representation of the patient's circulating blood (5).

 Tips from the Trenches: *To make vein relocation quicker, make a mental note of skin markers (moles, skin creases, freckles, etc.) on the skin above the vein when performing the initial survey. Loosen the tourniquet, assemble the equipment, put on gloves, and reapply the tourniquet. Locate the landmarks previously identified to facilitate vein relocation.*

Performing the Procedure

Step 1 ■ Put on gloves, tighten the tourniquet, and make sure all supplies are within reach. (See "Gloveless Phlebotomy and the BBP Club" in the Phlebotomy Tip of the Month section of the Appendices.)

Step 2 ■ Locate the preselected vein, and cleanse the site with 70% isopropyl alcohol. If the condition of the patient's arm necessitates excessive cleansing, several alcohol preps may be necessary. Allow the alcohol to dry. The drying process kills some bacteria and prevents the patient from experiencing a burning sensation on needle insertion. Blowing on the site is not recommended.

If blood cultures are being collected, cleanse the site with tincture of iodine, a solution of 1 % to 10 % povidone iodine or chlorhexidine gluconate according to facility policy. Allow the solution to dry and remove with an alcohol prep pad.

Once the site has been cleansed, do not touch the site. Repalpating for the vein after cleansing contaminates the site and risks infection. (It is estimated that nosocomial infections kill 75,000 patients every year [11]). If the vein's location has been lost and repalpation is necessary to relocate the vein, recleanse the site prior to the puncture.

 Tips from the Trenches: *OSHA regulations mandate that gloves be worn when drawing blood specimens for clinical testing.*

Venipuncture Using a Tube Holder (Figs. 3.6 to 3.11)

Step 3 ■ Place the first tube, stopper end first, into the tube holder without advancing it fully onto the interior needle. Remove the sheath from the needle and discard. (Note: OSHA prohibits resheathing needles [Box 3.5].) Inspect the needle for barbs or other imperfections. Replace needle if necessary. Grasp the holder with the thumb on top and two or three fingers underneath as shown. Rest the backs of the fingers firmly on the

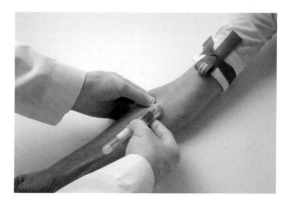

FIGURE 3.6 Anchor the skin from below by pulling the skin tight with the thumb of your free hand.

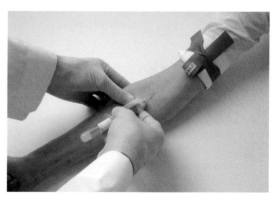

FIGURE 3.7 Insert the needle at an angle of 30 degrees or less.

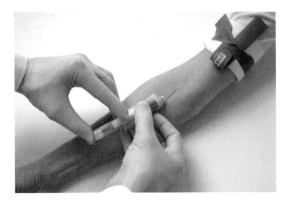

FIGURE 3.8 Apply the first tube.

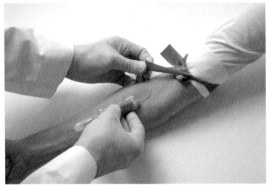

FIGURE 3.9 If possible, release the tourniquet when vein is accessed.

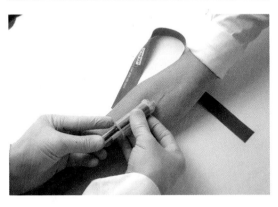

FIGURE 3.10 Remove and exchange tubes.

patient's forearm so that the bevel of the needle faces up and lies just off the skin at the intended puncture site. Grasp the holder at your fingertips with wrist turned so that the open end of the holder remains visible and accessible. This keeps the open end of the holder accessible for an unhindered exchange of tubes during the draw. Notify the patient of the imminent puncture (Box 3.6). A verbal warning is appropriate even if the patient appears unconscious or sedated. Do not assume that the patient is prepared for the puncture. Be aware that patients have varying degrees of sensitivity and pain tolerance.

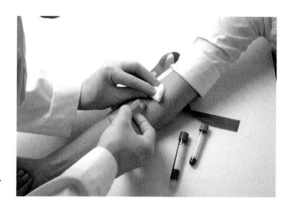

FIGURE 3.11 Apply light pressure, remove needle.

BOX 3.5 Recapping Needles

Historically, most accidental needlesticks occur when healthcare personnel recap a contaminated needle. Although needles with safety devices that prevent the necessity and ability to recap needles must be in use in healthcare environments, the potential still exists. According to OSHA, contaminated needles must not be recapped unless the employer can demonstrate that recapping is required or that no alternative is feasible (18). If no alternative is feasible, recapping must be done mechanically or by a one-handed method and justification for recapping must be documented in the facility's exposure control plan supported by reliable evidence (12).

It is undoubtedly easier for a facility to make sure sharps containers are available at the point of use and that employees are trained against recapping than to justify recapping to the satisfaction of inspectors. Providing for immediate disposal of contaminated sharps not only eliminates the uncertainty of acceptable justification, but more importantly, protects healthcare personnel from the uncertainty that comes with sustaining an accidental needlestick because provisions for immediate sharps disposal were not provided.

BOX 3.6 Notify the Patient

Notify all patients when the puncture is imminent, but avoid inflammatory phrasing, such as "this is going to sting" or "this is going to hurt." Instead, use more subtle phrases that are familiar, but not intimidating such as "poke," "pinch," "stick," or "mosquito bite."

It may be helpful to simulate the sensation on apprehensive patients by mildly pinching the skin at the intended puncture site to approximate the sensation. Patients should never be told they won't feel anything or that it won't hurt. Although it is possible to perform a painless venipuncture, a false representation can erode patient trust should the puncture be painful and can complicate the patient's next venipuncture.

Step 4 ■ Stretch the skin by pulling downward on the arm from below the intended puncture site, but not in such a way that it will obstruct the tube holder. When the skin is taut, the needle passes through it much easier and with significantly less sensation. This technique anchors the vein to prevent it from rolling away from the needle and minimizes the pain of the puncture. With a steady advance and a forward motion, guide the needle, bevel up, into the skin and the vein at an angle of 15 to 30 degrees (Figs. 3.12, 3.13). Advancing the needle too slowly increases the patient's discomfort while a rapid, jabbing motion can result in passing through the vein entirely.

 Tips from the Trenches: Healthcare personnel with both IV insertion and phlebotomy responsibilities have a tendency to raise the tip of the needle after it enters the skin during a venipuncture in an attempt to "pick up" the vein and thread the needle farther as they would in starting an IV. However, for blood collection, it is only necessary for the bevel to enter the vein. Once the upper wall of the vein is penetrated, all forward momentum stops and the needle rests in place while the sample is withdrawn. Any movement of the needle once it is within the vein is unnecessary.

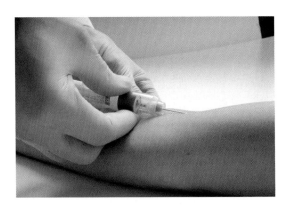

FIGURE 3.12 Insert needle at an angle of 30 degrees or less.

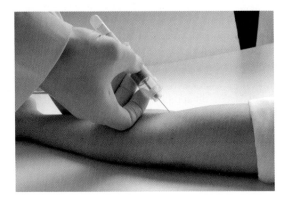

FIGURE 3.13 An excessive angle of insertion risks patient injury.

Step 5 ■ Once the needle is anticipated to be within the vein, release the skin and advance the collection tube fully forward in the holder so that the interior needle punctures the stopper of the tube. Maintain the position of the needle by resting it on the backs of the fingers holding the device on the patient's forearm for support. Use the flared wings of the tube holder to counteract the pushing pressure exerted on the bottom of the tube to maintain needle position. Pushing the tube forward without using these wings may drive the entire needle assembly forward, advancing the tip of the needle through the other side of the vein. To counteract the pushing pressure, position the index and middle finger on either side of the holder and push against the bottom of the tube with the thumb. Squeezing the thumb and fingers together advances the tube and pierces the stopper without disturbing the placement of the needle. Allow the tube to fill. The vacuum in the tube will pull blood from the vein and fill the tube to the appropriate level (see Box 3.7). Release the tourniquet once blood flow has been established

---

BOX 3.7   Minimum Fill Requirements

Laboratories that comply with the standards for laboratory testing have strict and well-defined specimen rejection criteria. One of the requirements that acceptable specimens must meet is that tubes with additives are filled to the proper level. Tube manufacturers calibrate the amount of additive in each tube to obtain accurate results based on a full draw. Underfilling tubes alters the optimal blood:anticoagulant ratio and can significantly affect test results and misrepresent the patient's actual physiology.

When a laboratory receives a specimen filled below the minimum acceptable volume, the specimen processor or testing personnel is obligated to request that another specimen be drawn. Failure to reject compromised specimens risks reporting inaccurate results and initiating a cascade of events that can affect the diagnosis, medication, and/or care of the patient. Collectors who submit underfilled specimens to the laboratory put the patient at risk when testing is delayed by the inevitable request for recollection. A far greater risk to the patient is when underfilled specimens are accepted and tested by unscrupulous testing personnel who fail to uphold minimum-fill standards.

Fortunately, many tests are not dependent on the tube being completely filled. Tubes without additives have no minimum fill requirements. Sodium citrate (blue stopper) tubes must be filled to at least 90% when submitted for aPTT testing (5). Minimum fill volumes for other additive tubes should be established and maintained by the testing facility in accordance with manufacturer's recommendations.

Some tubes are designed for a low-volume draw (i.e., difficult veins, draws on infants, children, or geriatrics, etc.) and contain a lesser vacuum and proportionally less anticoagulant. These "pediatric" or "partial-draw" tubes can be the same size and dimension as full-volume tubes, but will not fill to the same level. Some manufacturers place a line on the label of these tubes to approximate the optimum fill level. Submitting specimens filled below the established minimum volume for any tube is requesting that the laboratory compromise its testing integrity.

to prevent hemoconcentration from affecting the results if it is anticipated that the flow will not be interrupted (5).

Step 6 ■ If blood flow is not established, the tube may have lost its vacuum, the needle may be improperly positioned in the vein, or the vein may be too small for the size of the needle or for a vacuum-assisted draw. Follow the appropriate recovery technique as detailed in "Recovering the Failed Venipuncture," later in this chapter.

Step 7 ■ After the tube is filled, remove the tube without displacing the needle. To maintain needle position, grasp and pull the tube while pushing against the flared wings of the holder. If the tube contains an additive, gently invert it 5 to 10 times as soon as possible. If additional tubes are required, apply and remove subsequent tubes the same way, making sure they are filled in the proper order (see "Order of Draw," later in this chapter). Remove the last tube from the holder before removing the needle from the patient to prevent blood from dripping off the tip of the needle.

Venipuncture Using a Syringe

Follow Steps 1 and 2 from "Performing the Procedure."

Step 3 ■ Pull back on the plunger to unseat it from the barrel of the syringe, then push the plunger fully forward, expelling all air from the barrel. Remove the sheath from the needle. Inspect the needle for barbs or other imperfections. Replace needle if necessary. Grasp the syringe at the fingertips with the thumb on top and two or three fingers underneath as with a tube holder. This keeps the plunger accessible and the barrel of the syringe visible while filling. Position the needle with the bevel up just off the skin at the intended puncture site while resting the backs of the fingers holding the syringe on the patient's forearm for support. Inform the patient of the imminent puncture (Box 3.6).

Step 4 ■ Pull downward on the arm from below the intended puncture site with the thumb of your free hand from about an 8 o'clock position relative to the intended puncture site to stretch the skin. When the skin is taut, the needle passes through it with significantly less pain to the patient, reducing patient discomfort and anchoring the vein in place. With a steady forward motion, guide the needle into the skin and the vein at an angle of 15 to 30 degrees in one smooth motion. Advancing the needle too slowly increases the patient's discomfort while a rapid, jabbing motion can result in passing through the vein entirely.

Step 5 ■ Release pulling pressure on the skin. Once the needle is in the vein, it is no longer necessary to pull the skin taut or to anchor the vein. A visible "flash" of blood may appear in the hub of the syringe signifying the vein has been accessed. However, it is important not to consider this to be a reliable indicator. Many factors may prevent blood from entering the hub even though the needle is within the vein. Therefore, the absence of the visible flash of blood should not be interpreted as improper needle placement.

Step 6 ■ Pull the plunger back and withdraw an adequate volume of blood for the tests ordered. Push against the wings of the syringe while pulling back on the plunger to counteract the pulling pressure and maintain needle placement during the draw. Loosen the tourniquet once blood flow has been established to minimize the potential for hemoconcentration unless it is thought that doing so may risk completing the draw. Allow the syringe to fill. Be mindful that specimens drawn with syringes are especially vulnerable to clotting and require special consideration. The clotting process begins the moment blood enters the barrel of the syringe. During difficult draws, it may take a considerable amount of time to collect and transfer the specimen into the tubes. If this time exceeds 1 minute, significant clotting may take place within the syringe. If clots are small enough to go undetected they can alter the results without notice. Therefore, avoiding prolonged blood aspiration minimizes the effects clotting can have on specimen quality and results.

Step 7 ■ If blood is not obtained, the needle may be improperly positioned or the bevel of the needle may have attached to the upper wall of the vein. Since serious patient injury can result from needle relocation, manipulation of the needle should be conducted according to the Clinical and Laboratory Standards Institute recommendations. Follow the appropriate venipuncture recovery technique as detailed in "Recovering the Failed Venipuncture," later in this chapter.

 According to the Standards . . . when the vein is missed and needle relocation is required to salvage the venipuncture, lateral needle relocation in the area of the basilic vein is not permitted due to the close proximity of nerves and the brachial artery.

Using Winged Collection (Butterfly) Sets

Follow Steps 1 and 2 from "Performing the Procedure."

Step 3 ■ Assemble the set with a syringe or a tube holder as described in Chapter 2. If a syringe has been attached to the set, break the seal of the plunger by pulling it back to unseat it, then return it fully forward, expelling all air from the barrel. Remove the sheath and inspect the needle for barbs or other imperfections. Replace needle if necessary. Grasp the wings of the set, pinching them together between the thumb and index finger. Hold the device with the bevel facing up allowing the other fingers to rest on the patient's forearm and the needle to rest just above the intended puncture site at a low angle to the arm. Inform the patient of the imminent puncture (see Box 3.6).

Step 4 ■ Stretch the skin and anchor the vein by pulling downward on the arm from below the intended puncture site at about an 8 o'clock position relative to the intended puncture site so that the thumb does not interfere with needle insertion. Stretching the skin in this manner minimizes the pain of the puncture and stabilizes the vein to prevent it from rolling away from the needle upon insertion. Guide the needle through the skin into the vein with a steady forward motion keeping the angle at less than 30 degrees. Avoid a slow, timid puncture, which will increase the patient's discomfort. However, avoid a rapid, jabbing insertion, which will make passing entirely through the vein likely.

Step 5 ■ Release the skin after the needle is anticipated to be within the vein. Often, a flash of blood will appear in the line indicating venous access. However, do not rely on the flash of blood as an exclusive indicator because many variables, including low blood pressure, may prevent blood from entering the line.

Step 6 ■ Release the tourniquet as soon as the vein is accessed to minimize the effects of hemoconcentration unless doing so threatens the success of the venipuncture. If using a syringe, pull back on the plunger with gentle pressure using your free hand until a sufficient quantity of blood is obtained. If drawing through a tube holder, push each tube fully into the holder and fill in the correct order (see "The Order of Draw," later in this chapter), inverting each tube several times as it is removed.

Step 7 ■ If no blood is obtained while using a syringe, the needle may not be properly positioned in the vein or the pulling pressure on the plunger may be excessive causing the bevel of the needle to attach to the upper wall of the vein. If no blood is obtained using a tube holder, the tube may have lost its vacuum, the needle may be improperly positioned in the vein, or the vein is too small for the needle. (See "Recovering the Failed Venipuncture," later in this chapter,) Avoid side-to-side manipulation of the needle as this can permanently injure the patient.

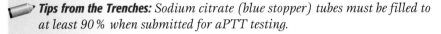 ***Tips from the Trenches:*** *Sodium citrate (blue stopper) tubes must be filled to at least 90 % when submitted for aPTT testing.*

Step 8 ■ After an adequate sample has been obtained, instruct the patient to unclench the fist. If the tourniquet is still applied, release it by pulling downward toward the puncture site, not upward toward the shoulder. Pulling it upward can cause the skin to pull away from the needle prematurely and the puncture site to bleed freely. Lay a 2- × 2-inch gauze lightly on the insertion point without applying pressure. (If the safety device activates within the patient's vein, perform the activation step according to manufacturer's instructions.) Remove the needle quickly, and then increase pressure on the puncture site. Activate the safety feature immediately according to manufacturer's instructions. Any delay in activation

It Could Happen to You

While inserting an IV, a nurse collected a syringe of blood from a patient. With the contaminated needle still exposed, she laid the syringe on the bed and taped down the IV tubing. Suddenly and unexpectedly, the syringe began to roll off the bed. Instinctively, the nurse reached for the device and the needle punctured the palm of her hand. She acquired hepatitis C from the exposure.

Question: What could the nurse have done to prevent herself from becoming infected?

Answer: Had the nurse activated the safety feature on the needle immediately upon removing it from the patient's vein, she likely would not have sustained a needlestick nor contracted hepatitis C. Vulnerability to a needlestick does not end until the contaminated needle is permanently sheathed or discarded into a sharps container.

increases the likelihood of an accidental needlestick. Studies show that 62% of all accidental needlesticks occur within moments of needle removal from the patient (14).

If blood was collected into a syringe, remove the needle from the syringe after assuring the device's safety feature has been activated, and attach a safety transfer device. Discard the contaminated needle. Do not remove the stopper from the tube and manually fill the tube. This may result in over-or under-filling. Insert the first tube to be filled into the device, advancing it onto the interior needle to puncture the stopper. Allow it to fill, bottom to top, without assistance to its stated capacity. Allowing tubes to fill top to bottom risks additive carryover. Fill each tube in the proper order of draw. (See "Order of Draw," later in this chapter.) If blood culture vials are to be filled, use a safety transfer device of the appropriate size to fit the vial. Invert tubes with additives several times immediately after filling.

It Could Happen to You

A nurse had just finished drawing blood into a syringe from a patient's subclavian central line. She held the tubes with one hand and pierced their stoppers with the conventional needle attached to the syringe instead of attaching a safety transfer device. While attempting to puncture one of the stoppers, the needle slipped off the cap and punctured her finger. She frantically scrubbed the puncture site, but a blood test several weeks later revealed that she had acquired hepatitis C.

Question: What could the nurse have done to prevent this accident?

Answer: Had the nurse drawn blood with a safety needle, she would have been able to activate the safety feature, remove the needle and attach a safety transfer device to fill the tubes. Tubes should never be filled from a syringe with the same needle used to draw the specimen.

According to the Standards . . . the use of cotton balls for applying pressure to the puncture site is discouraged. The cotton fibers can become imbedded in the fragile fibrin clot that forms at the puncture site and disrupt the plug when removed. Instead, apply pressure with gauze pads.

According to the Standards . . . it is the responsibility of the collector to apply adequate pressure to the puncture site. Bending the patient's arm at the elbow is not considered to be an effective means of applying pressure and should be avoided. Patients may be asked to assist, but the collector must be assured the helpful patient is applying adequate pressure. If inadequate pressure is applied, the collector may be responsible for complications including nerve injury, which can result from hematoma formation.

If the draw was performed using a tube holder, activate the safety device before or immediately after removing the needle from the arm according to manufacturer's instructions. Place the activated device directly into a sharps container. Any hesitation in disposal or safety feature activation puts the healthcare professional at risk of an accidental needlestick. Needle tube holder assemblies should be discarded as one unit. It is against OSHA regulations to remove the needle or to reuse the tube holder (15). In addition, studies have shown that tube holders become contaminated with trace amounts of blood even after one use (16,17). To properly protect healthcare personnel from accidental needlesticks, a sharps container should be available at the point of use. Use of needles without safety features is prohibited by OSHA (18).

Step 9 ■ Maintain pressure on the puncture site until bleeding has stopped. In patients who are on anticoagulant medication or aspirin, complete closure of the puncture site may be prolonged. Avoid the practice of bending the patient's arm at the elbow. This technique is not considered to provide adequate pressure and is discouraged by the Clinical and Laboratory Standards Institute (5) (Fig. 3.14).

Cooperative patients may be allowed to assist, however the collector is ultimately responsible for making sure adequate pressure is applied. Remove pressure and observe the insertion site long enough to assure that the puncture site has sealed. Observe for bleeding not only from the skin, but watch the tissue around the site for any raising or mounding that indicates the skin has sealed, but the puncture to the vein is still hemorrhaging (Fig. 3-15). If you suspect this to be the case, reapply pressure for several more minutes and check again. (See "Be Sure Before You Bandage" in the Phlebotomy Tip of the Month section of the Appendices.)

According to the Standards . . . patients should not be bandaged until the collector is assured that stasis is complete. This means bleeding must have stopped from not only the surface of the skin, but from the vein itself. Before

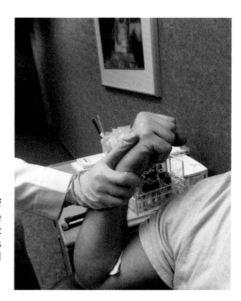

FIGURE 3.14 Avoid the practice of bending the patient's arm at the elbow. This technique does not provide adequate pressure and is discouraged by the Clinical and Laboratory Standards Institute.

bandaging, perform a two-point check: (1) check for superficial bleeding from the skin and (2) take a few moments to observe for bleeding from the vein into the tissue indicated by hematoma formation.

Step 10 ■ Specimens must be labeled properly and in the patient's presence without exception. Leaving the patient's side, without labeling the tubes completely and permanently, risks specimen misidentification and invites errors that can lead to patient mismanagement and death. (See "Label or Liable" in the Phlebotomy Tip of the Month section of the Appendices.)

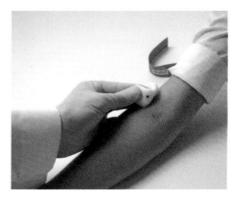

FIGURE 3.15 Observe for bleeding not only from the skin, but watch the tissue around the site for any raising or mounding that indicates the skin has sealed, but the puncture to the vein is still hemorrhaging.

Labeling specimens with abbreviated identifiers to facilitate complete labeling at a later time deviates from the established standards of the procedure and puts patients and healthcare personnel and their employers at great risk. Under no circumstances should specimen tubes be labeled before they are filled. Complete labeling includes the following entries:

- Patient's first and last names
- Unique identification number
- Date of collection
- Time of collection
- Initials of the individual performing the venipuncture

Many facilities have preprinted labels that contain proper patient information including the time the specimen is to be collected. Nevertheless, those who draw specimens must make a handwritten entry on the tube that includes the collector's initials and the actual time and date of collection. The same information must be entered in the permanent records. The time of collection is a critical element in the interpretation of many tests, including blood glucose and therapeutic drug monitoring.

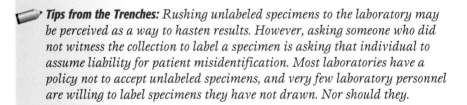 ***Tips from the Trenches:*** *Rushing unlabeled specimens to the laboratory may be perceived as a way to hasten results. However, asking someone who did not witness the collection to label a specimen is asking that individual to assume liability for patient misidentification. Most laboratories have a policy not to accept unlabeled specimens, and very few laboratory personnel are willing to label specimens they have not drawn. Nor should they.*

Step 11 ■ Bandage and thank the patient. Discard gloves and other waste in appropriate receptacles. For inpatient draws, return the room to its previous arrangement before leaving. If bedside trays, chairs,

It Could Happen to You

After drawing specimens from three inpatients, a lab technician left each room without permanently affixing the labels to each patient's specimen. Upon returning to the lab, she laid all the tubes on a counter and mislabeled the specimens. All three patients required blood bank testing. One of them, a 31-year-old wife and mother of four, received incompatible blood and subsequently died.

Question: How could this tragedy have been avoided?

Answer: Had the specimens been labeled at each patient's side, the mislabeling errors might not have occurred. Because improper labeling is potentially fatal, collectors must label all specimens completely and permanently before leaving the patient's side.

wastebaskets, bedside rails, and other items were moved, return them to a position that is convenient for the patient. Should the patient have to stretch or get out of bed to retrieve an item that has been displaced, a fall or injury could occur. Provide the patient with postvenipuncture care instructions according to facility protocol. (See an example of postvenipuncture care instructions in the Appendices.)

> *Tips from the Trenches: Some patients are allergic to the adhesive in bandages. If the patient indicates such an allergy, an alternative method should be used rather than leaving the site uncovered. For example, place a sterile 2- × 2-inch gauze over the puncture site, and apply a gauze wrapping around the circumference of the arm. Make sure the wrap is applied tightly enough to hold the gauze but not so tight so as to restrict circulation.*

Wash your hands and transport specimens to the laboratory. If the testing facility is off-site, process and store specimens according to the Clinical and Laboratory Standards Institute standards in regard to the effects of time and temperature on the tests to be performed (see Chapter 6, "Specimen Handling, Storage and Transportation"). Make no attempt to satisfy a patient's request for water, ambulation, lowering of the bed rails, etc., without checking with the patient's nurse or immediate caregiver to make sure that such actions are consistent with the patient's care plan and the physician's orders.

ORDER OF DRAW

Many blood collection tubes contain an additive to either facilitate or prevent the specimen from clotting. It is well documented that additive carryover from one tube to the next can occur and drastically alter results, leading to patient mismanagement (19–21). Additive carry-over occurs when the needle used to fill one tube transfers some of the blood/anticoagulant mixture from that specimen into the next tube filled. The anticoagulants and additives in some tubes can adversely affect results of tests performed on others. For example, lavender top tubes contain EDTA, an anticoagulant containing salts of potassium. If the tube filled after a lavender top tube is tested for potassium (i.e., a red, gold, speckle, or green top tube), any carryover of the blood/EDTA mixture from the lavender top tube to the next tube can introduce potassium and falsely elevate the potassium level in the tube that will be tested. The carry-over can be enough to make the patient with a normal potassium level appear dangerously high (hyperkalemic) and the patient with a dangerously low potassium level appear normal. In the latter case, the carry-over may prevent physician intervention with tragic results.

The order of draw can also impact coagulation studies such as protime (PT) and activated partial thromboplastin time (aPTT). If a minute amount of anticoagulant from a previous tube is transferred into a blue top tube used for coagulation studies, the introduction of the foreign anticoagulant can lengthen the clotting times. The falsely lengthened clotting time can lead physicians to misdiagnose the normal patient with a coagulation disorder or make the properly medicated patient appear overmedicated. In the latter case, the physician would be prompted to lower the patient's dosage inappropriately, making the patient vulnerable to stroke or cardiac arrest. Carry-over can also make an undermedicated patient appear well within therapeutic range risking the same potential outcome.

Violating the order of draw not only risks cross-contamination of anticoagulants, but can contaminate blood culture collections as well. The tops of blood collection tubes are not sterile. Therefore, the needles that puncture them are capable of picking up and transporting bacteria from one tube to the next. If the next tube is a blood culture bottle, the culture could be contaminated and lead the laboratory to report a positive blood culture on a patient who does not have a bacterial blood infection. Reporting positive blood cultures when the patient actually has a negative blood culture has been reported to significantly lengthen a patient's stay resulting in thousands of dollars of unnecessary tests and medication (22,23). Therefore, blood cultures must be collected before any other tubes are filled.

The order in which specimen collection tubes and bottles are filled can have a significant impact on patient results and how physicians respond to the results. Therefore, tube manufacturers and the Clinical and Laboratory Standards Institute have adopted a standard order in which tubes must be filled to prevent cross-contamination of additives or the bacterial contamination of blood cultures (5) (Table 3.2).

The order of draw is the same for using a tube holder as it is for drawing with a syringe. If only two or three tubes are to be collected, fill them as they fall within the recommended order. The Clinical and Laboratory Standards Institute no longer recommends drawing a discard tube when only a PT or aPTT is ordered because studies show no clinical significance in results obtained between first and second tubes (24–30). However, no studies have been published

---

TABLE 3.2 ▪ **The Order of Draw (5)**

1. Tubes or bottles for blood cultures
2. Tubes containing sodium citrate (light-blue stopper tubes for coagulation studies)
3. Serum tubes with or without clot activator or gel separator
4. Tubes containing heparin (green stopper tubes)
5. Tubes containing EDTA (lavender stopper tubes
6. Tubes containing sodium fluoride (gray stopper, etc.)

to measure the difference in specific factor assays (e.g., factor VIII) between the first and second tube drawn. Because coagulation studies have never been found to be affected, Clinical and Laboratory Standards Institute recommends that facilities adopt their own policy when drawing special factor assays (5). When used, the discard tube need not be completely filled.

 According to the Standards . . . a discard tube is not required when the citrate tube is the first or only tube drawn unless special factor assays are being collected (per facility policy) or when drawing through a winged collection set.

Even though studies negate the necessity of a discard tube prior to drawing routine coagulation tests, some facilities continue the practice as a precautionary measure. Follow the protocol established in your facility.

 According to the Standards . . . tubes must be filled in the recommended order to prevent erroneous results due to additive carry-over.

RECOVERING THE FAILED VENIPUNCTURE

When the vein is not immediately accessed, collectors can take limited measures to salvage the procedure (Fig. 3.16). There are several conditions that can prevent blood from entering the tube or syringe. These conditions depend on the equipment used.

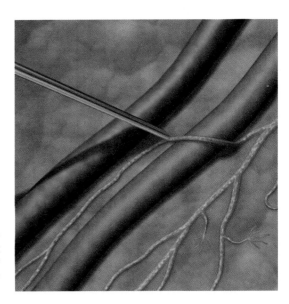

FIGURE 3.16 Improper needle relocation can inflict permanent nerve injury. (From the Center for Phlebotomy Education, with permission.)

If Using a Tube Holder

Cause: The tube may have lost its vacuum.

Resolution: Apply another tube.

Cause: The needle may not be positioned properly.

Resolution: Pull back on the needle slightly. If flow does not begin, continue pulling back farther until the bevel of the needle is just under the surface of the skin. If this fails, pull the tube within the holder back so that the inner needle no longer punctures the stopper and the vacuum is no longer applied. Repalpate for the vein. If located, reanchor the vein by pulling the skin down with the thumb of the free hand and move the needle deeper toward the vein. Be careful not to go so deep as to damage underlying structures. Excessive manipulation and side-to-side probing should be avoided (see Box 3.8).

Cause: The vacuum may be excessive, causing the vein to "collapse" or adhere to the bevel of the needle. This occurs if the diameter of the vein is too small for the vacuum within the tube.

Resolution: Apply a smaller tube of the same type or terminate the puncture and attempt a second puncture using a syringe and a 23-gauge needle with moderate pulling pressure.

BOX 3.8   Clinical and Laboratory Standards Institute Limits on Needle Manipulation

Strict limitations to needle relocation are necessary to prevent patients from injury. Because excessive needle relocation in the area of the basilic vein can damage nerves and the brachial artery (see "Phlebotomy Liability," Chapter 7), the Clinical and Laboratory Standards Institute places the following limitations on needle relocation when a blood sample cannot be obtained (5):

"Change the position of the needle. If the needle has penetrated too far into the vein, pull it back a bit. If it has not penetrated far enough, advance it farther into the vein. Rotate the needle half a turn. Lateral needle relocation should never be attempted in an effort to access the basilic vein, since nerves and the brachial artery are in close proximity. Try another tube to ensure the tube selected is not defective.

"Manipulation other than that recommended above is considered probing. Probing is not recommended. Probing is painful to the patient. In most cases another puncture in a site below the first site, or use of another vein on the other arm, is advisable.

"It is not advisable to attempt a venipuncture more than twice. If possible, have another person attempt to draw the specimen or notify the physician."*

---

*Reproduced with permission, from CLSI/NCCLS publication H3-A5-Procedures for the Collection of Diagnostic Blood Specimens by Venipuncture; Approved Standard-Fifth Edition (ISBN 1-56238-515-1). Copies of the current edition may be obtained from the Clinical and Laboratory Standards Institute, 940 West Valley Road, Suite 1400, Wayne, Pennsylvania 19087-1898, USA.

If Using a Syringe

Cause: Excessive pulling pressure on the plunger forces the vein to collapse onto the bevel of the needle.

Resolution: Reduce the degree of pulling pressure on the plunger. However, if the draw is prolonged, the specimen may hemolyze or clot within the barrel of the syringe before it can be transferred to tubes and render the specimen unacceptable. If the draw cannot be completed within 1 minute from the time blood first enters the barrel of the syringe, terminate the venipuncture.

Cause: The needle may not be positioned properly.

Resolution: While pulling back on the plunger, slowly withdraw the needle until it is just under the surface of the skin. If the needle originally went through the vein, this will salvage the puncture. If blood does not flow into the syringe, stop short of pulling the needle completely out of the skin and release the plunger so that the force of aspiration is no longer applied. Repalpate for the vien. If located, reanchor the vein by pulling the skin down with the thumb of the free hand and move the needle deeper toward the vein. Do not go so deep as to injure underlying structures. Pull back on the plunger. If blood flow is not established, terminate the attempt.

If Using a Winged Infusion Set

If a syringe is attached, follow the recovery instructions in the "If Using a Syringe" section of this chapter. Likewise, if a tube holder is attached, refer to the instructions in the "If Using a Tube Holder" section in this chapter.

Healthcare professionals who are unable to obtain a specimen after two punctures should allow a co-worker to attempt the collection. Repeated failures frustrate the patient, create anxiety, and erode the patient's confidence in the skill and professional judgment of the healthcare professional.

COMPLICATIONS

Fainting and Nausea

Specimen collection personnel must realize that all patients have the potential to faint during or immediately after a venipuncture, especially outpatients who are not recumbent. Watch for the signs of vertigo (dizziness) or syncope (fainting) and be prepared to protect the patient from falling. Pallor, perspiration, anxiety, lightheadedness, hyperventilation, and nausea can preempt a loss of consciousness. Make it a habit to ask patients if they feel all right, but don't rely on their answers totally, especially in the presence of any of the above symptoms. If the patient appears faint during the venipuncture, quickly release the tourniquet and remove the needle from the vein. Apply pressure to the puncture site and activate the safety feature of the collection device and/or dispose of the contaminated sharp immediately. Do not set a contaminated needle aside for later disposal even in light of the patient's circumstances. Maintaining the presence of mind and protecting yourself during a patient reaction is just as critical as caring for the patient. Do not attempt to walk a patient to a bed who demonstrates the signs of an impending loss of consciousness. Instead, lower the patient's head below the heart to increase the supply of oxygenated blood to the brain. Place a cold compress to the patient's forehead or to the back of the neck. Avoid the use of ammonia inhalants, which can induce respiratory distress should the patient be asthmatic. Call for assistance without leaving the patient's side. If a portable stretcher can be brought into the area, place the patient on it with assistance. Guard patients who experience fainting episodes until they have recovered completely, and document the incident according to facility policy.

Because inpatients are usually recumbent, they rarely experience vertigo or syncope. Nevertheless, being alert for the signs of vertigo or syncope is equally important, especially if the patient is drawn in a sitting position. If the symptoms appear, react as previously described. Request assistance if necessary.

Nausea may precede vomiting. Be prepared to offer nauseous patients an emesis basin. If vomiting occurs during the venipuncture, terminate the procedure immediately and allow the patient to recover. Delay specimen collection as long as possible to allow full recovery. Lay the patient on a cot or bed when recollecting the specimen. (See Chapter 7 for additional precautions.)

 According to the Standards . . . avoid using ammonia inhalants because asthmatic patients may develop respiratory distress.

Seizures

Patients who experience seizures during a venipuncture should be protected from injuries that may result. As with fainting patients, release the tourniquet, remove the needle from the vein, and immediately activate the device's safety feature. Apply pressure to the puncture site while restricting the patient's movements. Avoid firm restraint. Do not put anything in the patient's mouth during a seizure.

Hematoma Formation

Occasionally, blood will escape from the vein into the tissue during a venipuncture leading to a hematoma formation. Since hematomas exert pressure on nerves and can cause a permanent compression nerve injury and/or complex regional pain syndrome, rapidly forming hematomas should prompt the collector to terminate the venipuncture and apply adequate pressure. Hematomas that are allowed to develop not only risk injury and unsightly skin discoloration, but render the site unacceptable for future venipunctures because specimens collected from sites infiltrated with blood may be contaminated as the pooled blood decomposes and its by-products return to the circulation.

Hematomas can form under the following circumstances:

- When the needle penetrates the vein completely, and then is slightly withdrawn allowing blood to leak from the puncture to the underside of the vein
- When the vein is grazed during insertion and venous access is not achieved
- When the brachial artery is inadvertently punctured or nicked
- When the needle partially pierces the upper wall of the vein
- When the needle comes out of the vein before the tourniquet is released
- When drawing from fragile veins of geriatric patients
- When the needle selected is too large for the vein

Rapidly forming hematomas require immediate termination of the puncture. Slow, gradual hematoma formation, however, may be arrested without ending the venipuncture by releasing the tourniquet during the draw, thereby reducing the pressure within the vein. However, this may result in the cessation of the flow of blood into the tube or syringe. Collectors should give priority to minimizing hematoma formation over the collection of the specimen and be prepared to end a venipuncture prematurely if necessary.

Pain

Patients have varying degrees of pain tolerance. Patients who express intolerable pain should be asked if they would like the procedure to be discontinued. Patients who insist the needle be removed are withdrawing consent for the procedure. Their request must be honored.

Those who perform venipunctures must be able to differentiate between normal discomfort and pain that is unusual or excessive. Under no circumstances should a venipuncture be continued if the patient feels a shooting or electriclike pain radiating above or below the puncture site. Shooting pain toward the shoulder and/or hand indicates that a nerve has been provoked and demands the needle be removed immediately before permanent injury results. Failure to immediately remove the needle when the patient complains of a shooting, radiating, or electriclike pain distant to the puncture site not only risks permanent injury, but also subjects the collector and his/her employer to litigation. (See Chapter 7.)

 Tips from the Trenches: When patients feel a shooting pain sensation toward the shoulder and/or hand, it indicates that a nerve has been provoked and demands that the needle be removed immediately before permanent injury results.

IN THE LAB: HOW HEMOLYSIS ALTERS RESULTS

Hemolysis, or the rupture of red blood cells, usually occurs during specimen collection and is the most common reason laboratories reject specimens. For testing in which serum or plasma is required (e.g., red, gold, blue top tubes, etc.), hemolysis becomes evident by the red tinge it imparts to the liquid portion of the blood after centrifugation, varying in shade depending on the severity of red cell destruction. However, if the specimen collected is for a test that does not require centrifugation (e.g., CBCs), hemolysis usually goes undetected because the sample remains well mixed. Consequently, the results of the CBC can be inaccurate and present the physician with a vastly different hematologic picture of the patient.

Because hemolysis is the rupturing of RBCs, gross hemolysis alters results in two ways: (1) the physical destruction of red blood cells releases their contents into the serum or plasma; (2) the dilution of all components of the blood when the liquid content of the RBCs is released into the serum or plasma.

Test results that are falsely elevated because of hemolysis include: potassium, LDH, AST, ALT, phosphorous, magnesium, and ammonia. Values that are falsely lowered include RBC counts and hematocrit (3,13).

For specimens tested in facilities remote to the site of collection (i.e., long-term care facilities, clinics, physicians' offices without labs, home draws, etc.), collectors may not be notified that the specimen needs to be recollected for hours or even days after the draw. This underscores the importance of utilizing good technique while collecting specimens to minimize the potential for specimens to be recollected long after the patient has left the facility.

REFERENCES

1. Ernst D, Ernst C. *Phlebotomy for nurses and nursing personnel.* Ramsey, IN: HealthStar Press, 2001.
2. Berger D. Direct-to-consumer testing [Editorial]. *MLO* 2000;32:6.
3. Dale J. Preanalytic variables in laboratory testing. *Lab Med.* 1998;29:540–545.
4. Paxton A. Stamping out specimen collection errors. *CAP Today* 1999;13(5):1,14–16,18.
5. NCCLS. Procedures *for the collection of diagnostic blood specimens by venipuncture.* Approved Standard H3-A5, Wayne, PA; 2003.
6. Phelan S. Q&A. *Lab Med* 1999; 30:93.
7. Horowitz S. Venipuncture-induced causalgia: anatomic relations of upper extremity superficial veins and nerves, and clinical considerations. *Transfusion* 2000;40:1036–1040.
8. Becan-McBride K. Preanalytical phase an important requisite of laboratory testing. *Adv Med Lab Professionals* 1998;10:12–17.
9. Narayanan S. The preanalytic phase an important component of laboratory medicine. *Am J Clin Pathol* 2000;113:429–452.
10. Statland B, Bokelund H, Winkel P. Factors contributing to intra-individual variation of serum constituents: 4. Effects of posture and tourniquet application on variation of serum constituents in healthy subjects. *Clin Chem* 1974;20:1513–1519.
11. Berens M. Infection epidemic carves deadly path. *Chicago Tribune* 2002. July 21:1,8–9.
12. OSHA Compliance Directive 2-2.69. Available at: http://www.osha.gov/pls/oshaweb/owadisp.show_document?p_table=DIRECTIVES&p_id=2570 (accessed 1/17/05).
13. Becan-McBride K. Preanalytical phase an important requisite of laboratory testing. *Adv Med Lab Professionals* 1998;Sept. 28:12–17.
14. Centers for Disease Control and Prevention. Evaluation of safety devices for preventing percutaneous injuries among health-care workers during phlebotomy procedures. *MMWR Morbidity and Mortality Weekly Report* 1997;46:21–25.
15. Occupational Safety and Health Administration press release. www.osha.gov/pls/oshaweb/owadisp.show_document?p_table=NEWS_RELEASES&p_id=1285&p_text_version=FALSE (accessed 7/30/03).

16. Howanitz P, Schifman R. Phlebotomists' safety practices. *Arch Pathol Lab Med* 1994;18: 957–962.
17. Weinstein S, Hamrahi V, Popat A, et al. Blood contamination of reusable needle holders. *Am J Infect Control* 1991;19(2).
18. Occupational Safety and Health Administration. Occupational exposure to bloodborne pathogens: final rule. 29 CFR 1910.1030. *Federal Register* 1991;56:64003–64282.
19. Sun N, Knauf R. Cross contamination solved by technique. *ASCP Summary Report.* 1977;14:3.
20. Schaeffer J, Triplett D. Case history D: increased aPTT due to the presence of heparin. *Lab World* 1981;32:39–40.
21. Calam R, Cooper M. Recommended "order of draw" for collecting blood specimens into additive-containing tubes. *Clin Chem.* 1982;28:1399.
22. Bates DW, Goldman L, Lee TH. Contaminant blood cultures and resource utilization: the true consequences of false-positive results. *JAMA* 1991;265:365–369.
23. Schifman R. Editorial. *Mayo Clin Proc.* 1998;73:703–704.
24. Brigden M, Graydon C, McLeod B, et al. Prothrombin time determination: the lack of need for a discard tube and 24-hour stability. *Am J Clin Pathol* 1997;108:422—426.
25. Yawn, BP, Lodge C, Dale J. Prothrombin time: one tube or two? *Am J Clin Pathol.* 1996; 105:794–797.
26. National Committee for Clinical Laboratory Standards. *Collection, transport, and processing of blood specimens for testing plasma-based coagulation assays.* Approved Guideline, H21-A4. Wayne, PA, 2003.
27. McGlasson D, More L, Best H, et al. Drawing specimens for coagulation testing: is a second tube necessary? *Clin Lab Sci* 1999;12:137–139.
28. Gottfried E, Adachi M. Prothrombin time and activated partial thromboplastin time can be performed on the first tube. *AJCP* 1997;107:681–683.
29. Adcock D, Kressin D, Marlar R. Are discard tubes necessary in coagulation studies? *Lab Med* 1997;28:530–533.
30. Bamberg R, Cottle J, Williams J. Effect of drawing a discard tube on PT and APTT results in healthy adults. *Clin Lab Sci* 2003;16:16–19.

REVIEW QUESTIONS

1. According to the Clinical and Laboratory Standards Institute, the proper order of draw is:
   a. blood culture tubes or vials; sodium citrate tubes; serum tubes; heparin tubes; EDTA tubes; oxalate/fluoride tubes
   b. blood culture tubes or vials; serum tubes; sodium citrate tubes; EDTA tubes; heparin tubes; oxalate/fluoride tubes
   c. EDTA tubes; oxalate/fluoride tubes; non-additive tubes; sodium citrate tubes; serum tubes; heparin tubes; blood culture tubes or vials
   d. blood culture tubes or vials; serum tubes; EDTA tubes; oxalate/fluoride tubes; sodium citrate tubes; heparin tubes

2. It is important to draw sodium fluoride tubes as the last tube in the order of draw because carry-over of the anticoagulant can:
   a. alter red blood cell morphology
   b. facilitate clotting
   c. bind calcium
   d. contaminate blood cultures

3. Factors that can hemolyze a specimen during collection include:
   a. excessive probing, improper needle placement, excessive pulling pressure on the plunger of the syringe
   b. vigorous mixing of the specimen, drawing above an active IV, small needle size
   c. inappropriate blood:anticoagulant ratio, underfilling, prewarming
   d. drawing tubes in an improper order of draw

4. Blood tests that are falsely decreased in hemolyzed specimens include:
   a. LDH
   b. AST
   c. ALT
   d. RBC

5. Which of the following practices prevents hemolysis during venipuncture?
   a. drawing blood in the proper order of draw
   b. avoiding needles smaller in size than 23 gauge
   c. pulling quickly and firmly on the plunger of a syringe
   d. prewarming infant heels

6. The order of draw is established to prevent:
   a. hemoconcentration
   b. excessive anticoagulation
   c. underfilling tubes
   d. additive carry-over

7. Blue top tubes should never be filled after a tube that contains a different additive because:
   a. the needle can transfer a minute amount of anticoagulant from a previous tube into the blue top tube and cause erroneous results
   b. blue top tubes must be filled to 90% of the stated volume

    c. it can result in falsely lower potassium levels

    d. of bacterial contamination from the previous tube

  8. Underfilling an EDTA tube can result in erroneous results due to:

    a. incomplete anticoagulation

    b. hemoconcentration

    c. fibrin degradation

    d. excessive anticoagulation

  9. According to the Clinical and Laboratory Standards Institute, proper inpatient identification consists of:

    a. a nurse or other caregiver identifying the patient

    b. the patient stating his/her name, then comparing the information with the requisition(s)

    c. asking the patient to state his/her name, then comparing the information with the requisitions and the arm bracelet

    d. the patient confirming his/her name, then comparing the information with the requisition(s) and arm bracelet

10. The basilic vein's close proximity to the brachial artery subjects the patient to the potential for:

    a. paralysis

    b. an arterial nick and subsequent hemorrhage

    c. hemoconcentration

    d. Lymphedema

11. "Blind sticking," i.e., inserting a needle where veins are neither visible nor palpable, should:

    a. never be attempted

    b. be attempted only when no other veins can be located

    c. should be attempted only in the antecubital area

    d. should be attempted only with the patient's permission

12. The median cubital vein:

    a. typically lies in the center of the antecubital area

    b. typically lies in the median aspect of the antecubital area

    c. typically lies in the lateral aspect of the antecubital area

    d. runs in close proximity to the brachial artery

13. If the patient has had a mastectomy, punctures to the arm on the affected side are:

    a. permitted only with physician's permission

    b. permitted only if no other site is available

    c. permitted only if the mastectomy is more than 10 years old

    d. permitted only with the patient's permission

Difficult Draws, Alternative Sites, Pediatric Venipunctures

4

INTRODUCTION

A wide variety of patient conditions exist that challenge the skills of health-care personnel with blood collection responsibilities. This chapter discusses alternatives and special considerations when routine venipunctures are complicated by needle phobia, age, mastectomies, condition of the skin and veins, and intravenous (IV) therapy. Acceptable alternative sites in addition to the antecubital area are discussed, including their limitations. Finally, pediatric venipunctures are discussed with an emphasis on sensitivity to the emotions of children and the challenges they present.

After reading this chapter, the reader should be able to:

- Describe strategies for dealing with needle-phobic patients
- State the limitations on drawing blood from patients who have had mastectomies
- Explain the impact on specimen results when drawing from edematous sites
- Describe the limitations IV therapy imposes on site selection
- Discuss acceptable alternative sites when draws to the antecubital area are not possible
- Explain the proper procedure when drawing blood from a vascular access device
- Apply strategies to calm the fears of apprehensive children

DIFFICULT DRAWS

Needle-Phobic Patients

Anyone who has been drawing blood specimens for more than several months realizes that some patients have a paralyzing fear of needles. According to Dr. James Hamilton, a family practitioner in Durham, North Carolina and the world's leading authority on needle phobia, 20% of the population is needle-phobic (1). Those with needle phobia are thought to have a genetic predisposition to the condition. Experts estimate 80% of needle-phobics have a first-degree relative (parent, child, or sibling) with needle phobia (2). Although most avoid healthcare settings and prefer to let their health deteriorate, those who submit to blood tests require compassion and special care.

Experts on needle phobia urge those who collect blood specimens to recognize the signs of an individual with an extreme paranoia of needles and have a procedure in place that minimizes the trauma of the experience. Such patients usually demonstrate extreme apprehension in advance of a venipuncture or other needle event. One such patient was reported to have punched the phlebotomist and jumped out a second story window to avoid the venipuncture (1). Children with the condition will physically resist, cry, scream, and/or do anything within their means to avoid the event. (See "Calming Fears," this chapter.) When extreme apprehension is evident, healthcare personnel must recognize the patient as being needle-phobic and take measures to prevent the fear from becoming lifelong (Fig. 4.1). Such measures include:

- Applying an ice pack to the puncture site to prevent the patient from developing a shock reflex
- Using iontophoresis
- Administering sedating medication
- Applying topical anesthetics
- Demonstrating extreme compassion, patience, and understanding toward the patient
- Avoiding physical restraint as a substitute for compassion

Symptoms of the shock reflex that needle-phobic patients experience during a needle event include syncope (fainting), near-syncope, lightheadedness or vertigo on needle exposure, pallor, profuse sweating, and nausea. Patients who are needle-phobic often go into shock during or immediately after the procedure and develop arrhythmia, even cardiac arrest. At least 23 cases of death due to needle phobia are documented (2,3).

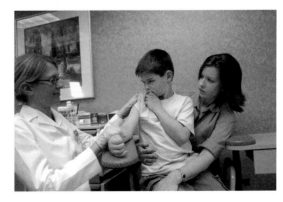

FIGURE 4.1 Healthcare personnel must able to recognize needle-phobic patients and take measures to minimize the trauma of the procedure.

According to Dr. Hamilton, the simplest, easiest method of preventing the shock reflex is to lay the needle-phobic patient flat with the legs raised and place an ice pack or ice cubes wrapped in a wet washcloth on the arm for 10 to 15 minutes before the draw. This numbs the arm and prevents triggering of the shock reflex. Some needle-phobic patients prefer to take sedating or calming medication a half-hour or so before the blood test. EMLA (Astra Pharmaceuticals/AstraZeneca, Switzerland), a topical anesthetic, can also be considered. However, depth of penetration is limited and the anesthetic must be applied by the patient to the proper site at least 1 hour before venipuncture. Use of pain medication should be documented and accompany the results.

One of the most promising techniques to treat needle-phobic patients is iontophoresis. Iontophoresis involves soaking a cotton pad with lidocaine and applying a tiny electric current for 10 to 20 minutes (Fig 4.2). The lidocaine numbs the venipuncture site completely to a depth down to the bone for at least 1 hour. An iontophoresis instrument must be ordered by a physician, but it is certainly easy and safe enough to be used by most healthcare personnel. (See Appendix for iontophoresis machines.)

Needle phobia experts agree that healthcare professionals must take a compassionate and sympathetic approach to patients that appear needle-phobic. They advise asking a series of probing but innocent questions to assess anxiety. Instead of bluntly asking "are you afraid of needles?" ask the following questions:

1. Have you ever had a blood draw or needle procedure before, and if so, did you have any difficulty with it?
2. Would you prefer me to hide the needle or keep it visible and explain everything I am about to do before I do it?
3. How can I make the procedure more comfortable for you?

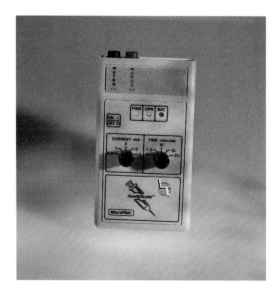

FIGURE 4.2 Needle Buster device. The Needle Buster delivers lidocaine into the skin by iontophoresis prior to venipuncture.

Tips from the Trenches: *Taking measures to minimize the trauma of a venipuncture is the key to averting a patient's lifelong paranoia to needles and a lifelong avoidance of medical care.*

When properly managed, the shock reflex that can occur during a needle event can be averted in those predisposed to the condition. Recognizing those with the potential and taking measures to minimize the trauma of the event are the keys to averting a lifelong paranoia and a lifelong avoidance of medical care. Most needle-phobic patients die prematurely from medical conditions that go untreated. Therefore, healthcare personnel who recognize needle-phobic patients and institute preventative measures and compassion can be personally responsible for not only relieving the suffering and anxiety during the venipuncture, but for prolonging the life of the patient.

Preventing Needle Phobia

Keith Lamb, confessed needle-phobe, has 15 suggestions for healthcare professionals to prevent those predisposed to needle phobia from developing the condition. They include:

- Put a mechanism in place to identify those children who are undergoing their first needle event. Suggest to physicians, especially pediatricians, that they ask their patients if it will be their first blood test and to notify the laboratory in advance of the patient's arrival.
- Survey parents and siblings to learn whether they may have exhibited needle-phobic reactions.
- Ask the parents whether the child has exhibited sensitivity to pain.
- Find out if the child has ever fainted upon exposure to fearful stimuli or has fainted for no known reason.
- If a vasovagal reaction is suspected or experienced during the first needle/blood exposure, all future needle events must be handled with an extra measure of compassion and understanding, and involve preventative measures. Future needle events should only be attempted in areas staffed by those trained in cardiopulmonary resuscitation and where a defibrillator is readily available.
- If associative fears are detected, professional behavioral therapy may be necessary prior to proceeding with any needle procedure.
- Those who are predisposed to needle phobia and undergoing their first needle event must have a painless experience. This justifies the prophylactic administration of topical anesthesia such as EMLA or iontophoresis. Let the patient's reactions be the guide as to if or when anesthesia can be reduced or eliminated.
- Healthcare personnel must not use negative emotional coercion, ridicule, or punishment for resisting fearful or painful procedures. Treat the cause of the resistance, not the resistance itself.

- A child should not be physically restrained or otherwise forced to undergo an elective needle event like a blood test unless it is required to save life, limb, or preserve long-term health. Even necessary procedures usually should not be forced on children with the possible exception of those patients who are mentally impaired or are so young that they are effectively unaware. When care is necessary for the very young or mentally impaired, medication (pharmacologic restraint) might be a better approach.
- Healthcare workers must be completely honest with parents and patients. There is no room for hiding the truth even if the intent is to be helpful. Painful procedures should not be untruthfully described as painless. When a patient experiences pain after being told a procedure won't be painful they feel confused, lose self-esteem, and ultimately become angry and distrustful. Many needle-phobics trace their lifelong distrust of healthcare workers to being lied to when they were young. Even euphemisms should be avoided such as "you might feel some pressure." Pressure and pain are different things; don't confuse them. While you should not exaggerate the discomfort, keep in mind that it is much easier to harm a child when using half-truths, untruths, and mistruths than by being honest about the procedure.
- If the child is too young to understand, then take steps to make needle events as painless and stress-free as possible until such time as they are mature enough to understand what is happening. A big helping of emotional support and praise goes a long way.
- Make it your goal to build the perception that health care is good and healthcare workers are friends. You know you are moving in the right direction when each encounter with the healthcare system is less stressful rather than more stressful. If the child is more stressed and expresses increasing resistance with each healthcare encounter, then you are moving in the wrong direction and you should stop and reassess your approach.
- Start by using anesthetic creams like EMLA (Astra Pharmaceuticals) so that the first procedure will be painless. During future visits, ask the child if and when they want to stop using the 'messy' cream or an iontophoresis machine. Be honest. Tell them it will hurt a bit, but for only for a few seconds. Tell them if it hurts too much, they can ask for the cream the next time.
- Give the child as much control as possible as soon as possible. It will serve them well for the rest of their life.

(Reprinted from *Confessions from a World Class Needle Phobe,* with permission. Available at http:///www.needlephobia.info.)

Age

Although every patient is different, each develops in stages related to his or her age. Patients have a wide variety of expectations based on many factors besides their age, including past experiences, physical and emotional limitations, cultural influences, likes and dislikes, and their value system (4). Understanding the implications of these factors is the key to becoming competent in drawing blood specimens from patients of a wide variety of ages.

Using techniques and strategies that are inappropriate for the age of the patient is likely to result in:

- A failed venipuncture
- Combative patients
- Customer service complaints
- Erosion of patient confidence
- Compromised specimens
- A lifelong fear of needles and/or healthcare facilities
- An unpleasant experience for phlebotomist and patient

Because each age group requires a unique approach to specimen collection, healthcare personnel with blood collection responsibilities should be well versed in the variations to approaching the patient and performing the procedure required for each age group with an emphasis on:

- Psychological impact of invasive procedures
- Communication skills
- Patient preparation and positioning
- Site selection
- Supplies and equipment
- Performance of the procedure
- Prevention of preanalytical errors
- Postvenipuncture care

While adult or geriatric patients are not likely to be apprehensive about a phlebotomy procedure, toddlers, children, and adolescents usually require an approach that is sensitive to fear and paranoia. (See "Needle-Phobic Patients," this chapter.) Being able to provide the comfort, assurance, compassion, empathy, and skill required to successfully obtain blood specimens from these younger groups is essential to all healthcare personnel with blood collection responsibilities.

Verbal communication skills are not critical with newborns and infants, but do contribute significantly to a positive experience with all other age groups. Speaking to a toddler requires simpler speech than speaking to an older child, while speaking to a geriatric patient must take into consideration the potential for hearing loss and dementia. For children, the purpose of effective communication is to secure cooperation. Use terminology that explains the nature of the procedure clearly and in terms that are not inflammatory, but reassuring (Fig. 4.3). For geriatrics, some of whom may be in early or advanced stages of Alzheimer's disease, the focus of communication is on making sure the patient can identify him/herself properly and knows what is happening.

Improperly preparing and positioning the patient can make a routine venipuncture on patients of any age difficult (Fig. 4.4). Regardless of age, the arm on which a venipuncture is being performed must be stabilized and supported. The patient must be prepared to anticipate needle insertion and maintain arm stability during the draw. Capillary blood is collected faster when

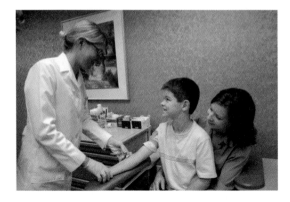

FIGURE 4.3 Healthcare personnel with blood collection responsibilities should be able to provide the comfort, assurance, compassion, empathy, and skill required to successfully obtain blood specimens from younger patients.

the puncture site is positioned below the plane of the heart, taking full advantage of gravity.

Selecting the site of the venipuncture is subject to many patient variables in addition to age. Nevertheless, hand veins often present more visible and palpable veins in newborns and geriatrics than in older children and adults. The equipment selected is a function of the site selected, but should take into consideration a dedication to reducing the discomfort of the procedure. For patients of any age who are sensitive to pain, especially children, the use of small-bore needles, such as 23-gauge, is recommended.

Although the basic venipuncture is performed similarly for all age groups, some age-specific variations exist. For example, draws on children require an assistant to assure the patient will not jump or jerk the arm away during the procedure. Adults and geriatrics who are familiar with the procedure and know what to expect rarely require such assurance. Although children require more patience and compassion, smaller needles to minimize discomfort, and a kinder touch than that required for adults, all age groups appreciate these qualities when subjected to a blood draw.

The potential for preanalytical errors to alter results during specimen collection varies from age group to age group. Newborns' and infants' skin puncture or incision sites require prewarming; adult draws require attention to all

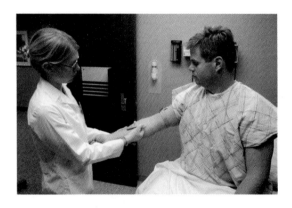

FIGURE 4.4 Improperly preparing and positioning the patient can make a routine venipuncture on patients of any age difficult and dangerous.

potential preanalytical errors including an improper order of draw, under-filled specimens, and prolonged tourniquet application; the same attention is required for geriatric patients as adults, but geriatric patients also require additional skill in needle placement and stability to prevent vein collapse and hemolysis.

Bandaging requirements vary from age to age. Bandaging is not recommended on newborns and infants, but is acceptable for older children and adults (Fig. 4.5). Geriatrics should be bandaged with consideration for skin that is far more delicate and susceptible to the adhesives in bandages than that of younger patients. (See "Capillary Blood Collection" and "Pediatric Venipunctures," this chapter.)

Mastectomy

During mastectomy, patients undergo the removal of lymph nodes, which control fluid balance (lymphostasis) in the arm on the same side and produce infection-fighting lymphocytes. Therefore, mastectomy patients have an increased susceptibility to infection and a painful, long-lasting fluid imbalance (lymphedema) when venipunctures and skin punctures are performed on the affected side. Because the fluid balance on the affected side of a mastectomy is compromised, blood drawn from the limb may be altered from that of the general circulation and may present the physician with misleading results.

Physicians are not in agreement on how long after a mastectomy the risk of lymphedema remains, making the decision to draw from the same side as a prior mastectomy physician-dependent. Therefore, drawing blood from an arm on the same side a mastectomy was performed should not be attempted without a physician's permission (5). This holds true for venipunctures and skin punctures/incisions, since both are capable of causing infection (6). Complicating site selection for those who draw blood specimens are patients who have undergone bilateral mastectomies. In such cases, a physician's permission must be obtained to draw specimens from either arm.

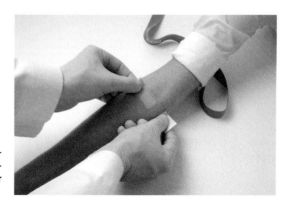

FIGURE 4.5 Bandaging is not recommended on newborns and infants, but is acceptable for older children and adults

Skin Injuries and Disorders

Specimens should not be drawn from sites that have been burned, scarred, or otherwise injured. Likewise, sites with rashes, bruising, inflammation, or infection should be avoided. Excessively bruised sites (ecchymoses) are not only more sensitive to puncture procedures, but blood obtained from them can be corrupt. As the body breaks down the hematoma, it returns the products of cellular degradation to the circulatory system, which can alter the composition of specimens drawn from the area.

Edema/Obesity

Blood should not be drawn from arms that are swollen from injury or fluids. The blood that circulates through such limbs may reflect the physiology of the affected limb, not of the patient in general. As a result, tests conducted on blood drawn from edematous sites can cause the physician to inaccurately assess the patient. Since the site from which specimens are drawn rarely accompanies the results, physicians trust that every specimen is drawn without site-specific interference or source of error. Drawing blood from edematous sites contributes to the potential for the patient to be managed according to compromised results.

Scarred and Sclerosed Veins

IV drug users and patients who have donated blood frequently may have scarred veins that make needle penetration difficult. Such veins lack elasticity and resiliency and should be avoided. Veins that are sclerosed due to disease or chemotherapy should also be avoided because they are difficult to access and may have impaired circulation.

Fistulas

A fistula is the surgical fusion of a vein and an artery near the surface of the skin with easy access for kidney dialysis procedures. Blood should never be drawn from a fistula since access may induce an infection necessitating reparative surgery. Because of the potential for complications, all draws to an arm containing a fistula should be avoided.

Heparin/Saline Locks

Heparin or saline locks provide venous access through which medications can be administered directly into the circulatory system. However, drawing blood specimens from heparin locks should be avoided if possible due to the potential for hemolysis and contamination of the specimen with heparin or saline. Drawing specimens through a heparin lock for coagulation studies should never be attempted.

IV Therapy

The selection of a venipuncture site on patients being infused IV fluids requires careful consideration. The infusion of fluids can significantly corrupt blood drawn from the same arm, drastically altering results and putting the patient at an extremely high risk should the test results prompt treatment, medication, or therapies (Fig. 4.6). To minimize the potential for infusing fluids to corrupt specimen results, collectors must carefully consider collection sites and techniques that prevent contamination. According to the Clinical and Laboratory Standards Institute (formerly NCCLS), whenever possible, venipunctures should be avoided on arms into which IV fluids are being infused(5). When this is not possible, draws below an active IV can be performed with adherence to a protocol designed to protect against specimen contamination.

 According to the Standards . . . draws from arms receiving IV fluids should be avoided whenever possible.

Drawing Below an IV Site

When no other alternative is available, collectors may draw below an active IV according to the following procedure (5, 7–14):

1. Shut off the IV for 2 minutes prior to the puncture with nursing assistance
2. Tighten the tourniquet below the IV site
3. Perform the puncture below the tourniquet as usual, discarding the first 5 cc of blood
4. Document that the puncture was performed below an active IV site

Drawing Above an IV Site

Fluids infusing in the hand, wrist, or forearm can corrupt blood specimens collected above the infusion site. The result is a diluted blood specimen that contains medications, electrolytes, donor blood, glucose, and/or other fluids

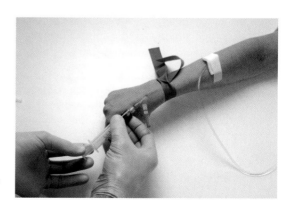

FIGURE 4.6 Drawing blood from the same arm as infusing fluids requires special consideration.

yielding laboratory results completely inconsistent with the patient's actual physiology. Attempting to trace the vein in which fluids are being infused with the intent to collect blood from another vein is not advised since the circuitous nature of the circulatory system makes such presumptions impossible.

 Tips from the Trenches: *Fluids infusing in the hand, wrist, or forearm can contaminate blood specimens collected above the infusion site.*

Some feel that temporarily interrupting an active IV prior to a draw above the infusion site is acceptable. However, collectors must not consider draws above an active IV unless facility policy permits this. Infused analytes can exist in higher concentrations above the IV for up to 24 hours after the IV has been shut off. Research shows that shutting off an IV for 3 minutes and drawing above the infusion site falsely elevated results if the analytes tested also existed in the IV fluid that was being infused (8,14). However, one study showed blood may be successfully drawn above a temporarily discontinued IV if the tests being drawn are not for coagulation studies, analytes that are being infused, and many other exceptions (15). According to the Clinical and Laboratory Standards Institute, facilities should carefully review the literature and establish their own policy.

If the facility allows specimens to be drawn above an active IV, exceptions must be well defined, extensively communicated, and applied without fail. Because the potential for error, miscommunication, and negative patient outcomes

It Could Happen to You

A nurse insisted the phlebotomist draw the patient's specimen above an active IV. The phlebotomist initially refused, but eventually drew the specimen when the nurse became adamant. The specimen was transported to the laboratory, tested, and found to have an extremely high glucose level. However, the draw site was not communicated to the laboratorian who ran the test and called the panic-level glucose to the floor. Because the nurse receiving the report was not the same nurse who insisted the specimen be drawn above the IV, she was unaware of the circumstances surrounding the draw and administered insulin. The patient died.

Question: How could this tragedy have been prevented?

Answer: If the phlebotomist resisted the nurse's intimidation and adhered to the policies of her department, the contaminated specimen would not have been drawn. In addition, if the draw site had been communicated properly to the testing personnel, the specimen would likely have been rejected or the results would likely not have been reported. Those who draw blood specimens must follow facility policy even when under fire. Facilities who allow specimens to be drawn above active IVs risk miscommunication and negative patient outcomes.

It Could Happen to You

The lab at a midsize hospital notified the nurse caring for a patient receiving heparin that the patient's PTT result indicated he was dangerously overmedicated. Following nursing protocol, she discontinued the patient's heparin therapy for 1 hour, then restarted it at a slower dose. Six hours later, a repeat PTT was drawn. This time the results showed that he was undermedicated. Questioning the validity of the earlier result, the nurse asked the patient where the phlebotomist drew the first specimen. He pointed to a recent puncture mark just above the IV.

Question: How could this medication error have been avoided?

Answer: In this case, the phlebotomist drew the first specimen above the active IV contaminating it with the heparin being infused. As a result, the patient's medication was unnecessarily decreased, making him vulnerable to stroke or other complications of blood clot formation. Had the phlebotomist drawn the specimen below the IV or from the other arm, the initial results would have been accurate and would likely have reflected a properly medicated patient, and the heparin therapy would not have been discontinued.

is greatly increased with such draws, facilities should carefully consider the risks of adopting such a policy. The risks increase in facilities at which specimens are drawn by nonlaboratory personnel because of the difficulty in managing a multiskilled work force. Should facility policy allow draws above active IVs, collectors must document the specimen was drawn above an existing IV

It Could Happen to You

Two days after surgery, a patient went into seizures. She was stabilized, stat blood tests were drawn, and she was moved into the intensive care unit. She died later that day. The physician accused the phlebotomist of drawing the stat blood work above the IV site. The physician claimed that had the specimen been drawn correctly he would have received accurate results and could have saved his patient's life. Upon investigation, the lab results from the draw did not support the accusation, and the phlebotomist was exonerated.

Question: Under what circumstances might the phlebotomist have been found to be responsible for the patient's death?

Answer: The stat lab work that was drawn showed the patient went into seizure and died because of dangerously low potassium and sodium levels. Although the results were inconsistent with the physician's charge that the blood was drawn above the IV site, had the phlebotomist not known the limitations to drawing above an IV and had actually done so, his role in the patient's death would have been difficult to deny. Knowing and applying the basic principles of blood collection are critical to immunize oneself against such charges.

and list the fluids being infused. Healthcare personnel should consider the following options before drawing a specimen above an active IV:

- Collecting the specimen by skin puncture—if the tests required can be performed on small quantities of blood, prewarming the patient's finger and performing a skin puncture can yield adequate specimen volumes. Consult with the physician about reducing the tests ordered to those that could be accomplished on blood collected by skin puncture.
- Drawing from a foot/ankle vein—such sites should only be considered with the physician's permission.

 Tips from the Trenches: *If the facility policy allows specimens to be drawn above an active IV, the site is never acceptable if the fluids being infused contain the analytes to be tested.*

Language Barriers

In our increasingly multicultural society, skills that overcome language barriers are becoming necessary in every facet of life. In healthcare, it presents unique challenges. Healthcare personnel with blood collection responsibilities need to communicate effectively to properly identify patients, address patient concerns, and assure that they understand the nature of the procedure. If necessary, seek the assistance of an interpreter so that the patient can be asked to state his or her name and to inform the patient of the imminent puncture in keeping with Clinical and Laboratory Standards Institute standards. (Fig. 4.7). If no interpreter is available to assist, specimen collection should not proceed until and unless proper patient identification can be made. Interpreters are also recommended to address common questions patients may have and to give postvenipuncture care instructions.

ALTERNATIVE SITES

In many patients, draws to the antecubital area are not possible for many reasons including:

- The inability to locate a suitable vein
- The infusion of IV fluids in or distal to (below) the antecubital area
- The antecubital area is excessively bruised from previous venous access procedures
- The presence of edema in the antecubital area
- Excessive scarring
- Skin conditions such as rashes, infections, burns, etc.
- Mastectomy
- Patient injury

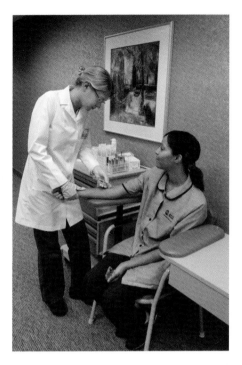

FIGURE 4.7 When drawing from culturally diverse populations, seek the assistance of an interpreter to properly identify the patient and to communicate effectively during the procedure.

In addition to the antecubital area, several secondary sites are acceptable for venipuncture. Healthcare professionals must carefully consider alternative sites and avoid the common misconception that any visible vein is acceptable for venipunctures. Drawing from unorthodox puncture sites without a comprehensive knowledge of superficial anatomy can increase the patient's risk of injury.

It Could Happen to You

A nurse went to the emergency department (ED) for postexposure evaluation and baseline blood work. The individual in the ED who drew the specimen attempted to access a surface vein on the anterior side of the wrist. Because of poor technique, she drove the needle deep into the tissue of the wrist, inflicting a permanent nerve injury that prevented the nurse from returning to acute care nursing.

Question: How could this injury have been prevented?

Answer: If the individual performing the venipuncture considered only acceptable sites for venipuncture, the injury would likely never have occurred. When coupled with poor technique, unorthodox puncture sites can be very unforgiving.

Acceptable alternatives to the antecubital area are the back of the hand; lateral side of the wrist, feet, and ankles (with physician permission); scalp veins (neonates); femoral arteries (physician only); and vascular access devices. Draws outside these sites must be approached with great trepidation and a thorough knowledge of the anatomy of the area and the risks involved.

Hand and Wrist Veins

When antecubital veins are not available, veins in the back or posterior side of the hand are usually the next veins considered. Veins here can be prominent and accessible for venipuncture, but are usually more delicate and smaller in diameter than the veins of the antecubital area. Therefore, the use of a syringe coupled with a 23-gauge needle or a 23-gauge winged blood collection set is recommended because the vacuum within collection tubes can collapse the veins. If a tube holder is used, tubes of a smaller volume, which exert a lesser vacuum to the interior of a hand vein, are preferred.

 Tips from the Trenches: When drawing veins on the back of the hand, use a syringe coupled with a 23-gauge needle instead of drawing directly into vacuum tubes, which can collapse the vein.

The hand veins of geriatric patients are typically very fragile and develop hematomas readily during or after the venipuncture. If a hematoma forms during the venipuncture, release the tourniquet immediately, remove the needle, and apply adequate pressure before bandaging. A second attempt may be made on the other hand, if accessible. Because geriatric patients often have compromised hemostasis (clotting processes), careful examination of the puncture site prior to bandaging and leaving/dismissing the patient is critical.

The hand veins of newborns and infants are small and delicate, but are often the only accessible veins.

It Could Happen to You

The staff of an office physician made five unsuccessful attempts to draw blood from the antecubital area of a patient during a routine office visit. The physician stepped in and attempted to access the patient's jugular vein and missed.

Question: Is the jugular vein an acceptable vein for venipuncture?

Answer: Definitely not. Unfortunately, physicians receive little if any training in phlebotomy. In this case, the patient was fortunate and did not sustain an injury from the failed jugular puncture. The patient was sent to the hospital laboratory where she was successfully drawn from the antecubital area in the first attempt. Had the physician inflicted an injury, he would have had difficulty justifying his choice of venipuncture sites.

In many patients without prominent antecubital veins, the best alternative site can be the vein on the lateral aspect (thumb side) of the wrist, which is often used to administer IV therapy. Like hand veins, this vein has a tendency to roll away from the needle when a puncture is attempted because it is not supported by tissue. Therefore, anchoring techniques are especially important to the success of punctures to the wrist and hand veins. The veins of the anterior (palm side) of the wrist and forearm should never be considered as an alternative site (5). The network of tendons and nerves serving the hand are precariously close to the surface of the skin. Punctures to this area risk patient injury.

 Tips from the Trenches: *Punctures to feet and ankle veins can lead to clot formation in patients who are prone to thrombosis or to tissue necrosis in diabetics.*

Veins of the Ankles and Feet

Venipunctures to the feet and ankles are acceptable on some patients. However, punctures to these veins can result in the formation of clots in patients who are prone to thrombosis or in tissue necrosis in diabetics. Therefore, before puncturing foot and ankle veins, make sure (1) the facility does not have a policy against such punctures, and (2) the physician has approved the site. Veins of the feet and ankles generally are small in diameter and require small-bore needles (22 or 23 gauge) in combination with a syringe.

Capillary Blood Collection

When blood cannot be obtained from the veins of the antecubital area or any of these secondary sites, it may be possible to obtain an adequate volume for testing from a skin puncture/incision procedure. Consult with testing personnel on the minimum volume required for the tests ordered. It may be necessary to consult with the ordering physician to reduce the tests requested to accommodate a skin puncture/incision in light of the difficulty in obtaining a venous specimen (see Chapter 5).

Vascular Access Devices

Vascular access devices (VADs) such as central venous catheters, arterial lines, and peripherally inserted central catheters (PICC) can provide direct access to the circulatory system without the necessity for venipuncture (Fig. 4.8). However, blood drawn through VADs is highly susceptible to contamination and prone to yield inaccurate results. Risks involved in drawing through VADs include:

- Increased likelihood of blood culture contamination
- Contamination of specimens with IV fluids
- High rate of hemolysis compared to venipunctures

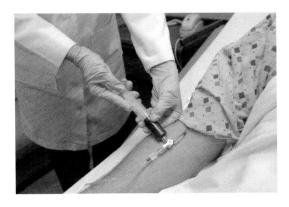

FIGURE 4.8 Blood drawn through VADs is highly susceptible to contamination and prone to yield inaccurate results.

- Potential to introduce air embolism into bloodstream
- Risk of introducing bacteria into bloodstream
- Risk of line occlusion

Because of these risks, blood collection personnel should avoid drawing from VADs whenever possible. Although the intent is to prevent the patient from the discomfort of a venipuncture, specimen contamination or hemolysis often results in recollection by venipuncture and delays in testing.

 Tips from the Trenches: *Drawing blood through vascular access devices risks contamination and is prone to yield inaccurate results.*

Care must be taken not to introduce bacteria or air into the patient's circulatory system during the collection process. Because of these and other risks to the patient and the specimen, it is imperative that draws through vascular access devices be performed only by healthcare personnel trained in the use and maintenance of such devices.

To prevent IV fluids from contaminating specimens, discarding a calculated volume of collected blood prior to obtaining an untainted specimen is required. The first few milliliters of blood withdrawn from VADs are contaminated with the infusing IV fluid. Therefore, it is important to discard an appropriate volume prior to obtaining the specimen that will be tested. The volume to be discarded depends on the "dead-space volume" of the VAD. The dead-space volume is the volume of fluid that the line can contain. The Clinical and Laboratory Standards Institute recommends discarding twice the dead space volume for noncoagulation testing and 5 cc of blood or six times the dead space volume for coagulation studies. As a rule of thumb, discarding 5 cc to 10 cc of blood from all VADs is usually adequate. Failure to discard the appropriate volume may result in contamination of the specimens and erroneous results. However, keep in mind the increased potential to induce anemia in young and geriatric patients that accompanies multiple sampling and excessive discard volumes. (See "Iatrogenic Anemia," this chapter.)

According to the Standards . . . The Clinical and Laboratory Standards Institute recommends discarding twice the dead space volume for noncoagulation testing and 5 cc of blood or six times the dead space volume for coagulation studies.

Blood drawn through VADs is also typically associated with a high frequency of hemolysis, i.e., the rupturing of red blood cells, which is difficult to prevent (13). Here's why: VADs are designed for the infusion of fluids, not the withdrawal of blood. Therefore, when blood is drawn through a VAD, it is being used for a purpose for which it is not intended. The shear forces that exist at the tip of the canula residing within the vein create turbulence when negative pressure is applied to withdraw a volume of blood. Such turbulence readily ruptures the fragile red blood cells, spilling the free hemoglobin within them into the liquid portion of blood. It is not until after the specimen is centrifuged in the laboratory that the extent of the hemolysis is evident, prompting testing personnel to reject the specimen since free hemoglobin interferes with the accuracy of most tests. (See "The Evils of Hemolysis," Chapter 5.) Hemolysis, therefore, is an inherent problem with vascular access draws and can be best prevented by avoiding draws through VADs whenever possible.

When no other alternative is possible, hemolysis may be minimized by drawing blood into a syringe instead of attaching a tube holder adapter and allowing the vacuum of the collection tubes to withdraw the sample. A syringe allows collectors to minimize the negative pressure, and therefore the turbulence, within the vein by pulling slowly on the plunger. After the syringe is filled with an adequate discard volume, the syringe is removed, discarded, and another one attached to the VAD. With gentle pulling pressure, obtain the specimen, remove the syringe, apply a safety transfer device to the syringe, and fill each tube in the proper order of draw. (See "Order of Draw," Chapter 3.)

Bacteria can colonize deep within indwelling lines and can be swept into blood being collected and inoculated into blood culture vials. As a result, the blood culture tests positive when the patient may not have a blood infection, and this can prompt the physician to administer unnecessary antibiotics and increase the patient's length of stay. (See "Blood Cultures," Chapter 5.) Although careful attention to aseptic technique can reduce contamination rates, to a large degree contamination is inherent to blood culture collection from VADs and cannot be prevented.

Studies Link High Hemolysis Rates with Emergency Room Draws

A study published in *Laboratory Medicine* concludes that specimens drawn by emergency department personnel have a higher rate of hemolysis than specimens drawn on the medical floor by laboratory-based phlebotomists. The report, "Hemolysis in Serum Samples Drawn by Emergency Department Personnel versus Laboratory Phlebotomists," was authored by researchers at Albert Einstein College of Medicine and the Montefiore Medical Center in New York, New York (16).

The study compared the hemolysis rates of blood drawn from emergency department (ED) patients by nurses or technicians (trained in the ED and without phlebotomy certification) versus samples drawn in nonemergency settings by certified phlebotomists. The hemolysis levels of blood drawn from 4,021 patients in the same acute care teaching hospital were assessed by technologists whose ability to visually detect hemolysis was standardized prior to the study. Only red top tubes used for chemistry studies were considered. The frequency of hemolyzed specimens drawn by ED nurses or technicians in the ED setting was found to be nearly eight times higher (12.4%) than those drawn by certified, laboratory-based phlebotomists from non-ED patients (1.6%).

In addition to certification and department affiliation, other variables include the venipuncture site selection, equipment used, mode of specimen transport to the lab, and the fill levels of the tubes observed for hemolysis. ED personnel predominantly drew blood distal to the antecubital fossa through plastic catheters, presumably in the lower forearm or back of the hand, whereas laboratory-based phlebotomists typically chose the antecubital area and used steel blood collection needles. The study also indicates that the ED department submitted partially filled tubes, which could have undergone hemolysis when sent to the laboratory through the hospital's pneumatic tube system. Specimens drawn by laboratory-based phlebotomists were hand-delivered to the lab.

The authors don't speculate which of the variables in the two study groups (equipment used, mode of specimen transport, partially filled specimens, prolonged tourniquet times, departmental affiliation, and phlebotomy certification) contributed most to the higher hemolysis rates observed in the ED group, but generalize that when all variables played out in their facility, specimens drawn by certified laboratory-based phlebotomists from the antecubital area were significantly less likely to be hemolyzed than specimens drawn by the personnel trained and the methods used in the ED.

It is unclear to the researchers just how much the ED personnel's practice of drawing through IV catheters contributed to the high hemolysis rates observed there. Using the Chi-squared analysis, hemolysis was significantly more frequent when specimens were drawn through vascular access devices by ED personnel than through metal venipuncture needles by laboratory phlebotomists. However, a logistic regression analysis found no correlation.

An article in the *Journal of Emergency Nursing* was more conclusive. According to the article, the study was inspired when the authors, all ED nurses and nurse educators, were told by the facility's lab manager that specimens coming from ED and drawn through IV catheters were excessively hemolyzed. The nurses disputed the lab manager's assertion and set up a comparative analysis of samples obtained in the ED through IV catheters versus venipuncture. The results confirmed the laboratory manager's assertion, showing that specimens drawn by nurses through an IV catheter were more than three times as likely to be hemolyzed than the specimens they drew by venipuncture (3.8% vs. 13.7%) (17). Ironically, the authors question their own results by referring to the "apparently higher hemolysis rates" in the discussion section of the report.

Nevertheless, the authors of the *Laboratory Medicine* article suggest that non-certified, nonlaboratory-based collectors tend to use equipment and techniques that skilled phlebotomists avoid as being associated with specimens of compromised integrity, that is, underfilling specimens, prolonged tourniquet time, draws outside the antecubital area, and drawing through IV catheters. They conclude that the best way to reduce pre-analytic hemolysis is to establish a standardized protocol for specimen collection. Many argue that such standardization is not possible without certification and a laboratory-based phlebotomy service.

(Adapted from *Phlebotomy Today*, 2002, vol 3, no. 9, with permission. Available at www.phlebotomy.com [accessed 10/17/2004].)

Femoral Artery

Draws from the femoral artery are usually required only in extreme circumstances (i.e., during CPR) and should only be performed by a physician.

Arterial Punctures

Arterial punctures should never be considered as an alternative to venipunctures when veins are difficult to find or access (5). The composition of arterial blood varies from venous blood in its concentrations of gases, cellular components, and other analytes (18). The arteries' increased blood pressure and close proximity to nerves require special skill and precautions. Arterial punctures for routine lab work (i.e., non-blood gas) should only be performed by physicians accessing the femoral artery under life-threatening circumstances as discussed under "Femoral Artery." Accessing the radial or brachial artery for non-blood gas testing is not an acceptable alternative to performing a venipuncture.

It Could Happen to You

A tech attempted to draw from a brachial artery for routine lab work and blood gases without an order. During arterial access, the patient violently jumped and flailed his arm causing the needle to slice the artery open. Because minimal pressure was applied, the patient bled profusely into his limb and required an emergency fasciotomy in which a muscle of his forearm had to be surgically removed, permanently disabling the patient.

Question: How could this injury have been avoided?

Answer: Invasive procedures such as venipunctures and arterial punctures should never be performed without an order. Had orders been given for routine lab work and arterial blood gases, separate punctures (i.e., a venipuncture and a radial artery puncture) should have been performed. After this patient's violent movement, adequate pressure should have been applied and the physician immediately notified to assess the damage to the brachial artery.

PEDIATRIC VENIPUNCTURES

Newborns and Infants

Specimen collection procedures on newborns and infants up to 12 months old require a great deal of expertise and a specialized phlebotomy technique. Because phlebotomy procedures and patient/specimen considerations are vastly different for this age group, only those properly trained should perform the procedure. Training should include considerations unique to this age group pertaining to:

- Pain reduction techniques
- Prewarming techniques
- Patient positioning
- Site selection
- Capillary versus venipuncture procedures
- Preserving specimen integrity
- Iatrogenic anemia
- Bandaging

The veins on infants in this age group are not well developed. Capillary specimens should be collected unless the physician specifically orders a peripheral draw (see "Capillary Blood Collection," this chapter). If a venipuncture is requested or required due to the volume of blood needed, veins of the hand may be more developed and accessible than those of the antecubital area. Draws to these veins must be done with a small gauge needle/syringe combination or winged collection set/syringe assembly. Assistance is required to stabilize the infant's hand and arm. Use the following procedure:

1. Identify the infant properly
2. Assemble equipment
3. Tighten a tourniquet, modified in size to fit around the infant's wrist or forearm
4. Have an assistant close the infant's hand into a fist and stabilize it to prevent movement
5. Locate the most suitable vein
6. If it is anticipated that venous access will take longer than 1 minute from tourniquet application, release the tourniquet to allow hemoconcentration to dissipate. Retighten after 2 minutes
7. Put on gloves
8. Cleanse the site
9. Perform and complete the venipuncture according to the procedure detailed in Chapter 3.

Because the veins of newborns are difficult to find, scalp veins are considered an acceptable site. However, draws to scalp veins are not to be routine and must only be performed by those properly trained in the technique. The use of a 23-gauge needle or winged collection set coupled to a syringe is preferred. Avoid the use of a 25-gauge needle because of its increased potential to hemolyze the red blood cells as they pass through the narrow opening of the bevel. Avoiding 25-gauge needles is critical, especially when an EDTA tube is the only tube being drawn. Since EDTA samples are not centrifuged, hemolysis goes undetected. As a result, the potential for erroneous results increases significantly.

 Tips from the Trenches: *In infants, hand veins may be more developed and accessible than those of the antecubital area.*

Iatrogenic Anemia

It is critical that blood volumes withdrawn on newborns and infants be minimal to prevent iatrogenic (hospital-acquired) anemia (Table 4.1). Because neonatal phlebotomy is highly specialized, many facilities employ specimen collection personnel specifically trained in neonatal phlebotomy.

TABLE 4.1 ▥ Maximum Blood Volume to be Withdrawn from Infants and Pediatrics

Patient's Weight (lb)	Patient's Weight (kg)	Maximum Amount to Be Drawn at Any One Time (mL)	Maximum Cumulative Amount to Be Drawn During a Hospital Stay of 1 Month or Less (mL)
6–8	2.7–3.6	2.5	23
8–10	3.6–4.5	3.5	30
11–15	4.5–6.8	5	40
16–20	7.3–9.1	10	60
21–25	9.5–11.4	10	70
26–30	11.8–13.6	10	80
31–35	14.1–15.9	10	100
36–40	16.4–18.2	10	130
41–45	18.6–20.5	20	140
46–50	20.9–22.7	20	160
51–55	23.2–25.0	20	180
56–60	25.5–27.3	20	200
61–65	27.7–29.5	25	220
66–70	30.0–31.8	30	240
71–75	32.3–34.1	30	250
76–80	34.5–36.4	30	270
81–85	36.8–38.6	30	290
86–90	39.1–40.9	30	310
91–95	41.4–43.2	30	330
96–100	43.6–45.5	30	350

(Reprinted from McBride K. *Phlebotomy Handbook: Blood Collection Essentials.* 6th ed. Upper Saddle River, NJ: Prentice Hall, 2003, with permission.)

According to the Standards . . . facilities should adopt a mechanism to monitor the volume of blood drawn for pediatric and critically ill patients to avoid phlebotomy-induced anemia.

Iatrogenic anemia refers to anemia induced by medical procedures, such as multiple phlebotomies. Increasing concern over the effects multiple sampling has on the quantity of circulating red blood cells has moved the Clinical and Laboratory Standards Institute to recommend that facilities monitor the quantity of blood withdrawn from geriatric and pediatric patients and other vulnerable patient groups (5). Most testing systems are now capable of performing complex test panels on minute quantities of blood. Therefore, some question the necessity for drawing specimens in volumes well in excess of that required for testing and encourage blood sampling to be performed using small-volume ("pediatric") tubes.

Monitoring sample volumes withdrawn from patients can be accomplished by the use of a log sheet kept in the patient's chart or near an infant's crib. Facilities should establish maximum blood volumes withdrawn per draw and per day based on the patient's weight and total blood volume (Table 4.1).

Exsanguinating Infants: Laboratories Seeking Limits

Concerns over excessive volumes of blood withdrawn from newborns and infants are prompting facilities to adopt policies to monitor total blood volumes that reduce the chance of phlebotomy-induced (i.e., iatrogenic) anemia. The removal of as little as 10 mL of blood from a newborn can result in up to a 10% depletion of the infant's total blood volume (19). Those subject to multiple sampling during the first week of birth are especially vulnerable to complications (e.g., severely jaundiced newborns).

Authors of a study published in *Pediatrics* concluded that phlebotomy overdraws were responsible for up to 15% of the packed cell transfusions given to very low birth weight infants (20). An article published in *Clinical Leadership & Management Review* reports a study conducted in Denmark showing blood losses from diagnostic sampling constitute up to 45% of the total blood volume of infants studied (21). Further, a study reported in *Laboratory Medicine* showed patients lose 4 mg of iron for every 10 mL tube of blood drawn (22). Therefore, not only do newborns and infants suffer from red blood cell depletion due to multiple sampling, but the risk of developing iron deficiency over time increases dramatically, increasing the impact of blood volume depletion.

According to the Clinical and Laboratory Standards Institute's document H3-A5, *Procedures for the collection of diagnostic blood specimens by venipuncture*, a mechanism should be developed to track the number of venipunctures and the volume of blood drawn for pediatric and critically ill patients to avoid iatrogenic anemia (5). The College of American Pathologists prompts volume considerations in its accreditation checklist by asking a question about the lab's review of "phlebotomy practices to minimize unnecessarily large blood draw volumes" (21).

Two publications suggest limitations on the volumes of blood to be collected from pediatric patients. The *Phlebotomy Handbook* contains a chart that places limits on quantities withdrawn per collection and per admission on pediatric patients from 6 to 100 pounds (2.7–45.5 kg). According to the authors, the recommended limit for an infant who weighs 6 to 8 pounds (2.7–3.6 kg) is 2.5 mL per draw and 23 mL per hospital stay of up to 1 month. A chart published in the Clinical and Laboratory Standards Institute Document H4-A5 shows that 10 mL of blood constitutes 7.9% of the total blood volume in a 1.1 pound premature infant (6).

Several sources provide assistance in establishing blood sampling limits based on body weight and estimating circulating erythrocyte volumes. For adults, blood volume can be calculated by applying the general assumption that a patient's average blood volume is equal to 70 mL per kilogram of weight (21). According to the Clinical and Laboratory Standards Institute, full-term neonates have a blood volume of 80 to 10 mL/kg, while the volume for premature infants is 115 mL/kg (6). Infant and children blood volumes range from 75 to 100 mL/kg.

Using these statistics, patients' circulating erythrocyte volumes can be calculated by multiplying the blood volume with the hematocrit. For example, a full-term infant weighing 2.7 kg (6 lb) has a total blood volume of 216 to 297 mL. Multiplying the more conservative volume (216 mL) with a typical newborn hematocrit (55%), the erythrocyte volume calculates to be 119 mL (216 mL × 0.55). If the facility caring for the infant adopts a policy not to withdraw more than 7% of any patient's total erythrocyte volume in any 24-hour period, a calculation of the maximum allowable whole blood volume that can be removed from the infant without extracting more than 7% of the RBCs can be made.

Blood volume withdrawn can be tracked with a log sheet attached to the infant's chart where phlebotomists and nurses can record volumes withdrawn. Blood volume withdrawn can also be tracked by recording volumes in laboratory records. Regardless, all mechanisms have the potential to break down if all who collect specimens in the facility don't comply.

Even with full compliance, however, tracking serves no purpose unless limits are established on volumes sampled and a protocol is adopted for situations in which those limits are met or exceeded. Unfortunately, no current guidelines exist in the literature, creating a challenge for facilities to develop and implement their own protocol. Such a protocol takes a coordinated effort between the laboratory and the nursing and medical staffs and must begin with thorough research on the current thinking about newborn and premature infant blood volumes and the degree of loss they can tolerate.

(Adapted from *Phlebotomy Today*, with permission. Available at www.phlebotomy. com/newsletter/Archives/0703.htm [accessed 08/25/03].)

Age: 1 to 3 Years

The antecubital veins of this age group usually are well developed. However, a fingerstick may be easier to perform because of a toddler's inability to remain still. But if a venipuncture is required to provide an adequate volume of blood for the tests ordered, a 23-gauge needle may be required by vein size and to ensure that the experience is as painless as possible.

Because of the active nature of this age group, recruit the assistance of a parent, guardian, or co-worker to stabilize the arm. Use only gentle, physical restraint to immobilize the arm during the venipuncture. For outpatients, position the child on the lap of the parent or guardian who can restrain the free arm of the child while an assistant immobilizes the arm to be punctured. If the parent is apprehensive about assisting or witnessing the procedure, escort him or her to a waiting area and position the toddler on a bed or cot with an assistant providing gentle restraint.

 Tips from the Trenches: *When drawing blood from toddlers, recruit the assistance of a parent, guardian, or co-worker to stabilize the arm.*

For inpatients, lay the patient, faceup, on a bed, crib, or cot with a parent or assistant providing gentle restraint to the free arm and to the wrist of the arm to be punctured. A second assistant may be necessary. The venipuncture can then be performed as outlined in Chapter 3.

Calming Fears

Conversationally, there is little that can be done to prepare children in this age group for a venipuncture other than being outwardly pleasant. Parent(s) or guardian(s) usually are present with patients in this group, whether inpatient or outpatient, and can be called upon to hold, comfort, and stabilize the child unless the facility has a policy against soliciting parental assistance. However, some parents prefer not to assist or even watch a venipuncture because the pain and distress it may bring to their child is more than they can bear. This apprehension should be recognized and accepted. Anxious parents should be allowed to wait outside the room while the procedure is performed with the help of a co-worker.

Age: 4 Years to Adolescence

By age 4, pediatric patients have well-developed veins in the antecubital area and usually pose little challenge to locating a suitable vein. It is essential that the arms of younger children in this age group be immobilized during the puncture to prevent unanticipated reactions. The older the child, the more likely the child will accept the procedure without incident. However, collectors should watch for signs of anxiety and apprehension in all age groups and seek the help of an assistant in stabilizing the patient's arm. A paralyzing fear can lurk just beneath the surface of composure, so prepare for all children to react unpredictably.

Avoid forcefully restraining a child who appears to be calm or only mildly anxious. Children don't like to be restrained any more than adults do. A firm, forceful grip can lead to increased anxiety and the loss of cooperation. Use only as much assistance as is necessary to assure the success of the procedure.

Calming Fears

A far greater challenge to healthcare personnel is to help the child overcome the natural anxiety that comes with an invasive procedure such as a venipuncture. Researchers suggest that up to 20% of the population has the tendency to become needle-phobic (see "Needle-Phobic Patients," this chapter). Some parents do an exceptional job preparing their child for a blood test, while others fail to address a child's natural anxiety for a needle event. To the child who has never experienced a venipuncture, fostering a realistic preconception is critical to a successful venipuncture and an uneventful experience. The preconception is often imbedded long before the patient comes to the facility. Overcoming a misperception of a venipuncture experience is one of the phlebotomist's greatest challenges.

For a child who has never had a venipuncture, one of their greatest fears is the fear of the unknown. All they know about how the procedure will feel is what they have heard from family and friends. If the source of their information has had a negative experience, the child will be led to expect the same. Sometimes the fear is insurmountable. Regardless of the child's perception and level of anxiety when presenting for a venipuncture, healthcare personnel trained to read apprehension and anxiety in their pediatric patients often can allay the fear in those who have been poorly prepared or have misconceptions of the procedure.

 Tips from the Trenches: *Healthcare personnel trained to read apprehension and anxiety in their pediatric patients can often allay the fear in those who have been poorly prepared or have misconceptions of the procedure.*

Approach all pediatric patients in this age group as if they have a deep, paralyzing fear, and work to calm and reassure them that the procedure does not cause the excruciating pain that they may have been led to believe. This takes a degree of compassion and patience that usually is not required for older children and adults.

 Tips from the Trenches: *Not everyone has the patience it takes to calm a child's fear of needles. Those without the skills to make a child's first experience uneventful should allow a co-worker with the patience required for successful venipunctures to perform the procedure.*

Start by establishing a rapport. Sit next to the patient, positioning yourself at the child's eye level so as not to project the intimidating effect of a towering, uniformed authority. Unless already conducted, an introduction is necessary. Ask the child if this is his/her first blood test. Regardless of the answer, talk the child through the procedure step-by-step, speaking in simple terms appropriate to the child's age. By explaining the procedure to the child (without showing the child the needle) fear of the unknown often dissolves as it becomes apparent to the child exactly what to expect. This technique is the single most effective way to turn an apprehensive child into a cooperative patient and takes less than 1 minute.

Demonstrate the use of the tourniquet by squeezing the child's upper arm with your hand, approximating the constriction the child will feel. Ask the child to make a fist. Be expressive and make light of the demonstration. When the child sees that you are not anxious, there is less of a reason for him/her to be anxious. Children also take their cues from their parents. If the parents are anxious about the procedure, give them the opportunity to wait outside the room. They often welcome the invitation.

Show the child the area of the antecubital where you will look for a vein and explain that you will cleanse the site with something "cold and kind of smelly." Recruiting the child's assistance gives him or her ownership in the procedure and helps to further calm apprehensions. Tell the child he/she has two jobs to do during the procedure. The first is to look the other way when told to. Explain that after looking away, he/she will then feel "a little pinch" or "something like a mosquito bite." Avoid the use of inflammatory terms such as "sting." Give the child an approximation of the sensation by gently pinching the antecubital area. This powerful tool—letting the child know exactly what to expect—can remove the last remnants of fear of the unknown. At that point, give the child the second job: to start counting to 10. Explain that by the time the child gets to 10, you will probably be done and will then put pressure on the site for a few minutes, you'll bandage it, and it will be over.

Never underestimate the power of bandages and stickers. To children, bandages are badges of courage that make everything all better. Stickers also have an appeal that gives the child something to look forward to when the procedure is over. Some facilities put stickers on a chart in full view of the outpatient drawing chair so that young patients can be preoccupied with selecting the sticker they want during the venipuncture procedure.

 Tips from the Trenches: *To children, stickers and bandages are considered badges of courage and honor that invite cooperation and serve as a reward for enduring a blood collection procedure.*

Despite your best efforts, some patients cannot be calmed. The fear may be so deeply ingrained from a prior experience or someone else's misperception that no degree of patience or compassion wins cooperation. Should anxiety escalate to a tantrumlike refusal, all hope for an uneventful experience is lost. If the child's parent(s) or guardian(s) are available and willing, their assistance may be necessary to restrain the child so that the procedure can be done quickly and without injury. Alternatively, solicit the assistance of one or more co-workers. Venipunctures should never be attempted on an uncooperative child without the assistance necessary to immobilize the arm and protect the patient and collector from injury. However, no degree of force used to restrain a patient should be so excessive that it could injure the patient. If the patient cannot be restrained without risking injury to the patient or collector, the physician should be notified of the difficulty in obtaining a specimen safely. Above all, follow your facility's policy on patient restraint.

In extremely anxious patients, obtaining the specimen by skin puncture/incision may be an alternative if the tests requested are minimal and require minute amounts of blood or serum (see Chapter 5).

 Tips from the Trenches: *When drawing blood from an uncooperative child, seek the necessary assistance to immobilize the arm and protect the patient and collector from injury.*

IN THE LAB

If a specimen is diluted with IV fluids, it will likely go unnoticed by the tech performing the test. Only the most grossly diluted specimens arouse suspicion. Therefore, it is dangerous to assume that contaminated specimens will be detectable during specimen processing or laboratory testing. If the patient has a normal blood level, a grossly diluted specimen can elevate or depress the test result to a level that would be viewed as life-threatening, prompting the physician to react with life-saving measures that may actually be life-threatening. Conversely, diluted specimens can yield negative or normal results when the patient's actual level is life-threateningly low or high resulting in inaction when intervention is crucial to the patient.

For example, let's say Mr. Smith, a new patient, has his blood drawn for a metabolic profile, toxicology screen, hepatitis profile, and CBC. The collector draws the blood above an active IV site unaware of the risks and limitations. When the specimen is sent to the laboratory for processing and distribution, processors immediately send the CBC tube to hematology and set the serum tube aside for clotting to complete (10 to 30 minutes). Once clotted, it is centrifuged for 5 to 10 minutes to separate the serum for the remaining tests.

The serum is removed and divided into three separate transfer tubes: one goes to the chemistry department for the metabolic profile, one to the toxicology lab for the toxicology screen, and the third to special chemistry for the hepatitis profile. Before the serum arrives in any of the other departments, the hematology technologist, having already tested the specimen, calls the physician with a hemoglobin of 5.9, which was confirmed by repeat testing. The physician responds by adding a type and crossmatch to the orders.

While the toxicology and special chemistry departments test their respective aliquots of serum, the technologist in the chemistry department has completed the metabolic profile and is now reviewing the results. The potassium level is 7.9—a level incompatible with life—and must be confirmed by repeat testing. Meanwhile, the toxicology lab has finished its testing and is reporting negative results on all metabolites. Mr. Smith is having his blood drawn again, this time for the type and crossmatch, a process that requires a special patient identification protocol that was not in place during the first draw.

Repeat testing of the potassium confirms the elevated level. The chemistry technologist notices that the glucose, sodium, and chloride levels also are significantly elevated. However, all other levels are well below normal or at the low end of the normal range. Because of the erratic results, the technologist calls the floor and discusses the results with the nurse. Together they make the connection between the elevated analytes obtained and the fluids being infused—D5W, KCl, and normal saline. Upon questioning, the collector admits that he drew the specimen above the IV.

It has been over an hour since the initial order was placed, and the physician has called the lab three times for the rest of the results. Mr. Smith is failing fast. The chemistry technologist investigates other tests ordered at the same time and alerts the hematology department, toxicology lab, and special chemistry section that the prior specimen was diluted and the results should be invalidated. The hematologist and toxicologist collaborate and notify the physician of the erroneous results. The physician puts the type and crossmatch on hold and orders a flurry of incident reports filled out. Mr. Smith's blood is collected a third time.

After processing, centrifugation, and distribution, the results from the fresh specimen eventually show normal hemoglobin, potassium, glucose, sodium, and chloride levels. All liver enzymes—previously at the low end of normal because of the dilution—are elevated. The toxicology screen is positive for alcohol and barbiturates and the hepatitis panel is positive for hepatitis B; all were initially negative from being diluted by the IV fluids.

Poor judgment in a specimen collection site initiated a cascade of actions, reactions, and delays that could have been prevented. Two additional collections, which would have been otherwise unnecessary; confirmatory testing; repeat testing; delays in treatment; and a blizzard of paperwork all translate into an expensive waste of supplies, equipment, and human resources. And that's not to mention the incalculable cost to Mr. Smith from the delay in treatment and diagnosis. Adding further to the total cost was the strain the incident placed on the relationships among the physician, the nursing department, and the laboratory.

REFERENCES

1. An interview with needle phobia expert, Dr. James Hamilton. *Phlebotomy Today* 2003; August. www.phlebotomy.com/archives/0803.htm (accessed 7/01/04).
2. Needle Phobia page. http://www.needlephobia.com (accessed 08/03/03).
3. What phlebotomists must know about needle phobia. *Phlebotomy Today* 2003;August. www.phlebotomy.com/archives/0803.htm (accessed 7/01/04).
4. Learn about age specific competencies. South Deerfield, MA: Channing L. Bete Co., Inc., 2000.
5. NCCLS. *Procedures for the collection of diagnostic blood specimens by venipuncture.* Approved Standard. H3-A5. Wayne, PA, 2003.
6. NCCLS. *Procedures and Devices for the Collection of Diagnostic Capillary Blood Specimens.* Approved Standard. H4-A5. Wayne, PA, 2004.
7. Dale J. Preanalytic variables in laboratory testing. *Lab Med* 1998;29:540–545.
8. Watson R, O'Kell R, Joyce J. Data regarding blood drawing sites in patients receiving intravenous fluids. *Am J Clin Pathol* 1983;79:119–121.
9. McCall R, Tankersley C. *Phlebotomy essentials,* 3rd ed. Baltimore, MD: Lippincott, Williams & Wilkins, 2003.
10. Hoeltke L. *Phlebotomy: the clinical laboratory manual series.* Albany, NY: Delmar, 1995.
11. Hoeltke L. *The complete textbook of phlebotomy.* Albany, NY: Delmar, 1994.

12. Kovanda B. *Multiskilling: phlebotomy collection procedures for the health care provider.* Albany, NY: Delmar; 1998.
13. Garza D, Becan-McBride K. *Phlebotomy handbook,* 6th ed. Upper Saddle River, NJ: Prentice Hall, 2002.
14. Read D, Viera H, Arkin C. Effect of drawing blood specimens proximal to an in-place but discontinued intravenous solution. Can blood be drawn above the site of a shut-off IV? *Am J Clin Pathol* 1988;90:702–706.
15. Savage R, ed. Q&A column. *CAP Today* 2002;16:102–103.
16. Burns E, Yoshikawa N. Hemolysis in serum samples drawn by emergency department personnel versus laboratory phlebotomists. *Lab Med* 2002;5:378–380.
17. Kennedy C, Angermuller S, King, R, Noviello S, Walker J, et al. A comparison of hemolysis rates using intravenous catheters versus venipuncture tubes for obtaining blood samples. *J Emer Nurs* 1996;22(6):566–569.
18. *Procedures for the Collection of Arterial Blood Specimens.* Approved Standard. H11-A4, NCCLS. Wayne, PA, 2004.
19. Becan-McBride K, Garza D. *Phlebotomy handbook.* Upper Saddle River, NJ: Prentice Hall, 2002.
20. Lin JC, Strauss RG, Kulhavy JC, et al. Phlebotomy overdraw in the neonatal intensive care nursery. *Pediatrics* 2000;106:E19.
21. McPherson R. Blood sample volumes: emerging trends in clinical practice and laboratory medicine. *Clin Leadership Mgmt Rev* 2001;15(1):3–10.
22. Q&A. Blood volumes needed for common tests. *Lab Med* 2001;4:187.

REVIEW QUESTIONS

1. The ideal gauge of needle for children, hand veins, and small surface veins is the:
   a. 20 gauge
   b. 22 gauge
   c. 23 gauge
   d. 25 gauge

2. If a patient refuses to be drawn, you should first attempt to:
   a. use physical restraint
   b. explain the importance of the tests
   c. cancel the tests
   d. ask your department head or supervisor to draw the specimen

3. All of the following practices will calm the anxious patient except:
   a. exuding confidence
   b. collecting tubes in their proper order
   c. explaining the procedure beforehand
   d. being pleasant and compassionate

4. Blood obtained through vascular access devices (VADs) are associated with:
   a. collapsed veins
   b. elevated iron levels
   c. hemolysis
   d. infection

5. The Clinical and Laboratory Standards Institute recommendation for drawing from vascular access devices is to:
   a. have the nurse shut off the IV for 2 minutes, tighten the tourniquet below the IV, and draw the specimen, discarding the first 5 cc of blood
   b. discard twice the dead space volume for noncoagulation testing and 5 cc of blood or 6 times the dead space volume for coagulation studies
   c. discard six times the dead space volume for noncoagulation testing and 5 cc of blood or twice the dead space volume for coagulation studies
   d. release the tourniquet for two minutes to minimize hemoconcentration

6. The simplest, easiest method of preventing a needle-phobic patient from experiencing a shock reflex is to:
   a. sedate the patient prior to the venipuncture
   b. administer oxygen to the patient during the procedure
   c. perform a fingerstick instead of a venipuncture
   d. lie the patient flat with the legs raised and place an ice pack on the arm prior to the draw

7. Drawing blood from an arm on the same side a mastectomy was performed:
   a. should not be attempted without physician's permission
   b. can be performed if there are no other alternatives
   c. can be performed with patient's permission
   d. can result in hemolyzed specimens

8. According to Clinical and Laboratory Standards Institute facilities should establish maximum blood volumes withdrawn per draw and per day on newborns and infants according to:
   a. the patient's age
   b. the patient's weight and total blood volume
   c. facility protocol
   d. *Clinical Practice Guidelines* from the National Association of Neonatal Nurses

9. Accessing the radial or brachial artery for non-blood gas testing:
   a. is not an acceptable alternative to performing a venipuncture
   b. is an acceptable alternative to performing a venipuncture
   c. should only be performed when the femoral artery is not accessible
   d. is only acceptable with patient permission.

10. When collecting specimens from _____, assurance that a venipuncture procedure does not cause excruciating pain requires compassion and patience.
    a. adults
    b. newborns
    c. geriatrics
    d. children

11. Shutting off an IV for 2 minutes and drawing above the infusion site:
    a. is acceptable when no other site is available
    b. can falsely elevate results if the analytes tested also existed in the IV fluid that was being infused
    c. is acceptable only when accessing a vein other than the one with the IV
    d. can be performed without nursing supervision

Special Collections: Arterial, Capillary, and Blood Culture Collection

5

INTRODUCTION

Besides venipuncture, three other vascular access procedures in phlebotomy require special skills and training: arterial punctures, skin punctures, and blood culture collections. In this chapter, the techniques unique to these specialized procedures will be discussed.

Upon completing this chapter, the reader should be able to:

- Detail the procedure for drawing capillary specimens
- Describe the proper procedure for drawing arterial blood gases
- Discuss the differences in commonly tested analytes between arterial and venous blood
- Describe the Modified Allen test
- Identify the common causes of contaminated blood cultures
- Discuss ways to reduce blood culture contamination rates
- Describe the proper procedure for preparing a site for blood culture collection

CAPILLARY BLOOD COLLECTION

Capillary specimens contain a mixture of blood from capillaries, venules, arterioles, and tissue fluid. Performing skin punctures/incisions instead of venipunctures significantly minimizes the risk of injury to the patient. However, the difference in the concentration of several analytes in capillary specimens is clinically and/or statistically significant (1).

- Glucose (higher)
- Potassium (lower)
- Total protein (lower)
- Calcium (lower)

Obtaining blood specimens by skin puncture or incision can be an alternative to venipuncture on patients for whom venous access is difficult when minute quantities of blood are sufficient for testing (Fig. 5.1). On newborns, skin puncture/incision is preferred over venipunctures because of the difficulty in obtaining blood by venipuncture and because of the hazards that venipunctures pose to infants, including blood volume depletion (1).

Although fingerstick glucose monitoring is the most common application of skin puncture techniques on adults, technologic advancements are making testing on a few drops of blood possible for a growing number of tests. Those applications for which skin puncture/incision may be advantageous include (1):

- Severely burned patients
- Extremely obese patients
- Patients with thrombotic tendencies
- Geriatric or other patients in whom superficial veins are very fragile or not accessible
- Patients performing tests at home
- Point-of-care testing
- Newborn testing
- Patients with a paralyzing fear of needles

Keep in mind that due to the sensitivity of fingertips, skin punctures can be more painful than properly performed venipunctures. Like venipunctures, without consideration for the effects of preanalytical errors on test results, blood can be significantly altered during the collection process and mislead the physician into mismanaging the patient. Strict adherence to the principles and techniques of skin puncture/incision procedures is essential to minimize the potential for error and negative patient outcomes.

Equipment

Puncture devices should be designed for single-use and contain a retractable, spring-loaded point or blade to prevent accidental needlesticks (Fig. 5.2). Nonretractable lancets or devices that necessitate the manual removal of the sharp after use put the collector at risk for an accidental needlestick and must not be used.

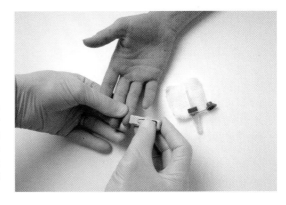

FIGURE 5.1 When minute quantities of blood are sufficient for testing, obtaining blood by skin puncture or incision can be an alternative to venipuncture on patients for whom venous access is difficult.

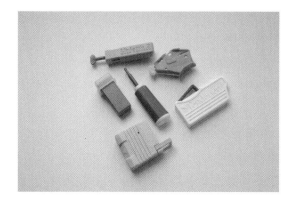

FIGURE 5.2 Puncture devices should be designed for single-use and contain a retractable, spring-loaded point or blade to prevent accidental needlesticks.

 Tips from the Trenches: The use of manual lancets or blades without a retractable feature is a violation of the Occupational Safety and Health Administration (OSHA) regulations.

 According to the Standards . . . when selecting the appropriate depth of puncture to the fingers of older children and adults, consult test requirements and the recommendations for usage from the device's manufacturer.

There are two styles of capillary blood collection devices: incision devices and puncture devices. Incision devices slice through capillary beds in varied depths and lengths; puncture devices, also known as lancets, penetrate vertically into the tissue in varied depths. Many styles and varieties of each are available. However, incision devices are less painful than lancet devices and require fewer repeat incisions and shorter draw times than lancet devices (2,3). This is especially critical for infant heelsticks.

Puncture devices are preferred for patients who require frequent sampling of minute quantities of blood, for example, self-monitored or bedside glucose testing. Because puncture devices penetrate and incision devices lance, sites that are repeatedly punctured can be used more frequently than sites that are lanced.

Other capillary sampling equipment includes:

- Alcohol preps
- Gauze pads
- Gloves
- Microcollection containers
- Sharps container
- Bandages
- Newborn screening cards
- Plastic capillary tubes
- Capillary tube sealer

Site Selection

The location of the puncture must be carefully considered in addition to the patient's age, accessibility of acceptable sites, and the tests ordered. Careful consideration must be given to the depth of the puncture with regard to the site selected. The thickness of the tissue on the side of an infant's heel can be as little as 2.0 mm and 1.0 mm at the posterior curvature of the heel (1).

Therefore, heel punctures on infants must never be performed on the back of the heel, and, when performed on either side of the heel, must be no deeper than 2.0 mm. The thickness of the tissue on the fingers of children and adults varies significantly. Refer to manufacturer's recommendation and facility policy when selecting the appropriate skin puncture/incision device for older children and adults.

Birth to 12 Months

For newborns and infants up to 12 months of age, only punctures to the medial or lateral (inner and outer) plantar surface of either heel are acceptable (Fig. 5.3). Depth of penetration should not exceed 2.0 mm. Avoid punctures to excessively bruised or traumatized sites, as the specimen obtained will likely be contaminated as the circulation clears the blood from the tissue and returns the breakdown products to the bloodstream. The arch of the sole and the back curvature of the heel should also be avoided; the tissue in these areas is thinner than that at the sides of the heel. Punctures to the fingers of infants in this age group are not acceptable due to the risk of bone penetration and the complications that can ensue, including infection and gangrene.

1 Year to Adult

For patients 1 year of age and older, capillary blood is typically collected from the fleshy pad of the third or fourth finger only. The thumb should be avoided

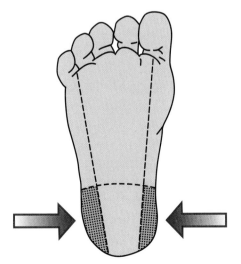

FIGURE 5.3 Sites for heel punctures on newborns and infants up to 12 months are limited to the medial or lateral plantar surface of either heel. (From McCall RE, Tankersley CM. *Phlebotomy essentials,* 3rd ed. Philadephia: Lippincott Williams & Wilkins, 2003.)

TABLE 5.1 ■ Acceptable Sites for Capillary Sampling (2)		
	Acceptable Sites	**Areas to Avoid**
Newborns and infants up to 12 months	Medial or lateral sides of the heel	Fingers of newborns All other areas of the foot including the arch and posterior curvature of the heel
Older children and adults	Fleshy pads of the third (middle) or fourth (ring) finger	Thumb, index, and pinky fingers; earlobes

because its skin is often too thick and callous. The second or index finger can also be callous and is significantly more sensitive than the other fingers and also should be avoided. Finally, avoid punctures to the fifth finger (pinky) as its flesh is not thick enough to ensure that the bone will not be pierced. Fingersticks should not be performed on the sides of the finger, but on the fleshy pad because the flesh on the sides is only half as thick as the flesh on the pad, increasing the risk of bone penetration (4). Other areas to avoid include the earlobe and swollen, infected, or excessively bruised sites (Table 5.1).

Procedure

Preparations for a skin puncture/incision are similar to those for a venipuncture. Observe standard precautions, identify the patient properly, ensure the test requirements are met (e.g., fasting, time of collection, etc.), and cleanse the site as described in Chapter 3. The use of a tourniquet is not required or recommended.

Prewarming

Prewarming the anticipated puncture site for a few minutes with a warm compress or cloth has multiple benefits. When the capillary beds are warmed, the flow of blood through the area increases sevenfold (1). If using a warm wash cloth, make sure the temperature of the compress does not exceed 42°C (Fig. 5.4). Warmer temperatures may burn delicate neonatal skin. Commercial

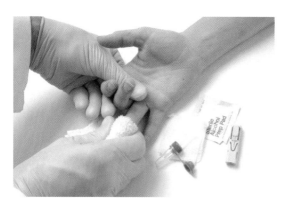

FIGURE 5.4 Prewarming the heel or finger increases the flow of blood through the capillary beds sevenfold.

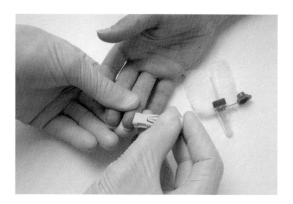

FIGURE 5.5 Performing the puncture or incision.

infant heel warmers are available that warm to a limited temperature when activated. Either method works well when applied for 3 to 5 minutes prior to the puncture. Gently massaging the site also helps to increase circulation. When properly prewarmed, specimens are obtained quicker and require little if any tissue compression, which contaminates the specimen with tissue fluid and hemolyzes red blood cells. Prewarming skin puncture/incision sites, therefore, is the single most effective way to ensure that the test results will accurately reflect the patient's physiology.

Perform the Puncture/Incision

Wash hands and put on gloves. Place the puncture or incision device on the cleansed skin with minimum skin compression. Pushing the device forcefully onto the tissue closes the distance between skin and bone and risks bone penetration (Figs. 5.5 through 5.8).

When performing the procedure, position the device to cut perpendicular to the lines of the fingerprints, not parallel with them, to prevent blood from "channeling" away from the collection device (Fig 5.9). Activate the triggering mechanism of the device and remove it from the skin. Discard the device into an appropriate sharps container. Since the first drop of blood contains

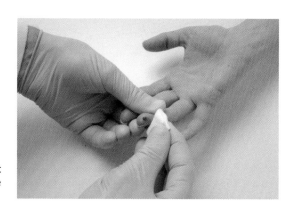

FIGURE 5.6 Wipe away the first drop of blood with a clean gauze pad.

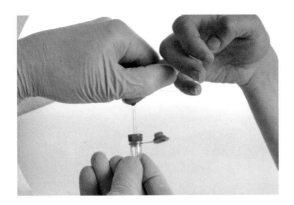

FIGURE 5.7 Collecting specimen into tube. Allow the specimen to fill the tube.

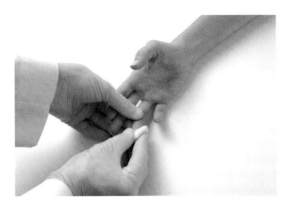

FIGURE 5.8 Applying pressure.

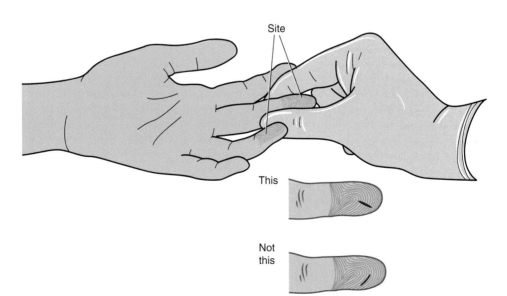

Site

This

Not
this

FIGURE 5.9 Perform the puncture perpendicular to the lines of the fingerprint, not parallel to prevent blood from "channeling." (From McCall RE, Tankersley CM. *Phlebotomy essentials*, 3rd ed. Philadelphia: Lippincott Williams & Wilkins, 2003.)

tissue fluid released by the trauma of the puncture, wipe away the first drop of blood with gauze to avoid diluting and contaminating the specimen. Allow subsequent drops of blood to freely flow into the collection tube. When using a bedside testing device such as a glucose meter, apply the specimen to the test strip or the appropriate testing interface. It may be necessary to gently squeeze the fingertip or heel to facilitate an adequate flow of blood. However, avoid excessively "milking" the site. Squeezing the tissue increases the likelihood that the red cells will rupture (hemolyze) and contaminate the specimen with tissue fluid. If excessive squeezing is required because of an inadequate blood flow, the procedure should be terminated and an attempt made on another site after prewarming.

When more than one collection tube is required for testing, follow the proper order of draw established by the Clinical and Laboratory Standards Institute (formerly NCCLS) (1).

Order of Draw for Capillary Specimens

1. Lavender top (EDTA) tubes for blood counts
2. Tubes with other additives
3. Tubes without additives

This order is necessary to prevent platelets from clumping together and to obtain accurate CBC results from the EDTA tube. When the puncture is performed, platelets rush to the site and adhere not only to the breaks in the vascular walls, but also to each other. If the EDTA tube, which is used to provide a platelet count to the physician, is collected late in the draw, platelets are more likely to adhere to each other in the specimen, making accurate platelet counts unlikely. Other additive tubes (if required) are filled after the EDTA tube to minimize the potential for clotting that could occur in the specimen during the collection process.

Allow blood to flow freely into the tube by gravity and/or capillary action. Position the finger or heel on a plane below that of the heart to further facilitate an adequate blood flow. Elevating the puncture or incision site serves to minimize the flow of blood through the area. Also, orient the puncture or incision site vertically downward so that it faces the floor. This allows blood to flow directly into the collection tubes instead of running down the finger or heel to reach its lowest point. When the blood flows freely from the capillaries into the collection tube, less sample is lost to the skin and collecting the sample is less likely to require a "scooping" technique, which can force tissue fluids into the specimen.

Tubes with additives should be periodically mixed during collection with a gentle tapping of the collection tube on a hard surface to prevent coagulation. Alternatively, tap the side of the tube with your finger. (Note: Caution should be taken when collecting blood into an open tube system because excessive agitation can allow aerosols and droplets to escape. Therefore, appropriate personal protection equipment should be worn according to facility protocol.)

Fill all tubes according to the manufacturer's minimum fill requirements for all tubes that contain anticoagulants. If collecting blood directly into capillary tubes or microhematocrit tubes, fill the tube two-thirds to three-fourths full and seal with the appropriate sealing compound immediately. Only plastic or Mylar-coated microhematocrit tubes should be used.

Once an appropriate volume of blood has been collected, apply pressure with gauze to the puncture site. Seal and mix the collection tube(s) with gentle inversion. It is of paramount importance that before the specimen leaves the patient's side it is labeled properly with the patient's name, identification number, date and time of collection, and the initials of the collector as specified in the facility's policy. Multiple microhematocrit tubes can be identified by attaching a label around them collectively, like a flag, and placing them inside a large test tube for transport.

When bleeding has stopped, bandage the patient according to facility policy. For older children and adults, it is less critical to bandage a skin puncture/incision site than to bandage a venipuncture site, and this may be left up to the patient. Bandaging neonates and infants less than 2 years old, however, is not recommended for two reasons: (1) young skin is much more sensitive to the adhesive over time and (2) bandages pose a risk of ingestion and/or airway obstruction should they become displaced (1).

Before leaving the patient or allowing outpatients to leave, remove and discard gloves and all supplies and equipment from the area. This is especially important when collecting blood from infants in cribs and car seats. Wash your hands and transport the specimen to the testing facility with consideration given to the effect that time, temperature, and delays in processing will have on test results.

Neonatal Screening

Today, all newborns are screened for a battery of metabolic and congenital disorders. The tests that comprise the battery vary from state to state and must at least include phenylketonuria (PKU) and hypothyroidism by federal law. Additionally, some states test for galactosemia, sickle cell disease, HIV, and homocystinuria, maple syrup disease and other congenital disorders, and inborn errors of metabolism. When collecting specimens for neonatal screening, drops of blood are allowed to absorb freely onto absorbent paper and allowed to dry before transport to an approved testing facility.

1. When entering the nursery, follow facility protocol for washing hands, wearing a gown, and identifying the infant.
2. Do not allow the collection tray to come in contact with patient surfaces. To protect against the spread of nosocomial infections, place the tray on the floor or protect the surface with paper or cloth towels or diapers that can be removed upon exiting the nursery.

3. Identify the infant. Crib cards are not an acceptable form of identification and should not be relied on to be accurate. Compare the information on the infant's identification bracelet with the newborn screening requisition and screening card. If there is any discrepancy or the bracelet is missing, notify the nurse or immediate caregiver. Do not collect any specimen until the infant's identity is confirmed or the discrepancy is resolved.

4. Prewarm the infant's heel for 5 to 10 minutes with a warm cloth not to exceed 42°C. Alternatively, commercial infant heel warmers are available and can be used. Massaging the heel while prewarming also increases the blood flow through the capillary beds and facilitates specimen collection.

5. Cleanse the site with isopropyl alcohol or the appropriate disinfectant according to facility protocol. Alcohol has been identified as a threat to the integrity of neonatal skin by the Association of Women's Health, Obstetric and Neonatal Nurses and the National Association of Neonatal Nurses in a published Clinical Practice Guideline (5). According to the guideline, isopropyl alcohol is discouraged because of drying to the skin. Povidone iodine or chlorhexidine is preferred, but should be removed after the procedure to minimize absorption. However, the manufacturers of some chlorhexidine products advise against using the agent on infants less than 2 months old.

6. Perform the puncture with a disposable, retractable heel incision device or lancet. Avoid previously punctured sites and sites that are bruised or in which the skin is otherwise compromised. Immediate repeat punctures with a second device should not be performed.

7. Allow a free-flowing drop of blood to accumulate, then touch it to one of the printed circles of the newborn screening card. Repeat for all circles. Allow the specimen to completely saturate the paper to the other side. Do not collect additional drops onto the same circle. Do not fill the circle from both sides. If inadequate blood flow prevents proper specimen collection, repeat the procedure on the opposite side of the heel or on the other heel.

8. Apply pressure to the site with a gauze pad until bleeding has stopped. Do not bandage the site. Adhesives damage the delicate skin of newborns and can become a choking risk should they be dislodged.

9. Remove all testing supplies and equipment from the area.

10. Complete the information requested on the card and submit to the appropriate testing facility after allowing the sample to dry.

Often, specimens for neonatal screening are rejected because of inadequate specimen collection. To facilitate accurate results and prevent the trauma of unnecessary re-collections, adhere to the requirements of the testing facility. It is imperative that all the circles of the neonatal screening card are filled from one side of the paper and completely saturated on both sides of the paper. Underfilled circles or cards can result in an inability to perform all the tests required by law.

ARTERIAL PUNCTURES

Concentrations of oxygen and carbon dioxide in arterial blood provide valuable information on the body's acid-base balance and the ability of the lungs to exchange oxygen. Therefore, arterial blood provides information to the physician not otherwise available. Typically, arterial blood is analyzed for pH, carbon dioxide (PO_2), oxygen (O_2), bicarbonate (HCO_3), base excess, and oxygen saturation. Some clinical instruments used to measure these arterial analytes are also capable of reporting the concentration of analytes typically obtained from venous specimens. This versatility negates the necessity for a separate venipuncture when arterial blood gases are ordered at the same time as tests routinely performed on venous blood. The composition of arterial blood compares favorably with that of venous blood with the following exceptions (4,6):

- pH
- The concentration of gases
- Bicarbonate
- Ammonia
- Glucose
- Lactic acid
- Alcohol
- Packed cell volume

Healthcare personnel whose responsibilities include arterial puncture for blood gas analysis recognize the unique skills necessary for this procedure. Comprehensive training beyond simple venous access procedures is necessary and should include detailed instruction on anatomy, respiratory physiology, arterial site selection and preparation, preanalytical errors, and the complications of arterial access.

An arterial puncture should never be performed as an alternative to a venipuncture when venous access is difficult (Fig. 5.10) (7). Performing an arterial puncture risks patient injury to a greater degree than a

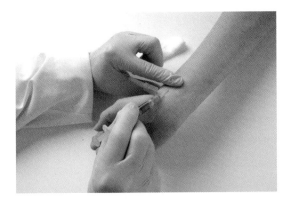

FIGURE 5.10 An arterial puncture should never be performed as an alternative to a venipuncture when venous access is difficult.

venipuncture and should never be performed without a physician's written permission.

 According to the Standards . . . arterial punctures should never be performed as an alternative to a venipuncture when venous access is difficult.

Acceptable Sites

Three sites are acceptable for arterial access: the radial, brachial, and femoral arteries (Fig. 5.11). The preferred site is the radial artery due to its accessibility and the ability of the ulnar artery to provide collateral circulation to the hand, keeping it oxygenated, should complications arise during or after radial artery access. The radial artery is readily accessible in most patients and has the advantage of being close to the surface of the skin. This not only simplifies locating and accessing the radial artery, but also makes it easier to apply

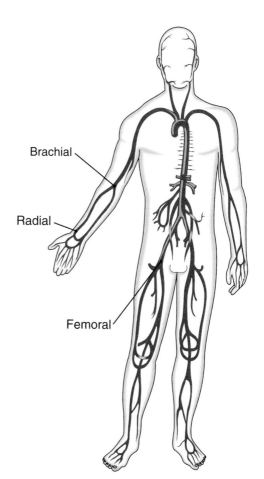

FIGURE 5.11 Three sites are acceptable for arterial access: the radial, brachial, and femoral arteries. (From McCall RE, Tankersley CM. *Phlebotomy essentials,* 3rd ed. Philadephia: Lippincott Williams & Wilkins, 2003.)

pressure after the puncture is complete to prevent hematoma formation, which can lead to nerve injuries and other complications.

To locate the radial artery, apply pressure with the index and middle fingers to the lateral aspect of the patient's wrist and feel for a pulse. If possible, hyperextend the patient's wrist. This brings it closer to the surface of the skin, anchors it in place, and stretches the skin for ease of needle insertion. The radial artery should lie close to the surface of the skin in the fossa between the tendon and radius of the lower forearm near the wrist. Locating the pulse may be difficult in obese patients or patients with low blood pressure or a weak pulse. Before considering a brachial artery, the presence of a radial artery should be assessed in both wrists to reduce the risk to its lowest possible degree. The brachial artery should be considered only after determining neither radial artery can be safely and successfully accessed.

When the radial artery is not accessible, assess both brachial arteries for the most accessible choice. The brachial artery is larger and usually has a stronger pulse than the radial artery. However, it is not supported by tendons and bone like the radial and lies in close proximity to the basilic vein and median nerves, which can be inadvertently pierced during a brachial access procedure. In addition, its depth makes it difficult to apply adequate pressure once the needle is removed, increasing the risk of the complications of hematoma. The brachial artery can be located by applying pressure with the index and middle fingers to the fossa between the muscles of the upper arm in the medial anterior aspect of the antecubital area just above the elbow. Feel for the presence of a pulse.

When brachial access is not possible, for example, during CPR, an arterial specimen may be obtained from the femoral artery. This procedure should only be performed by a physician or emergency personnel specifically trained in femoral access procedures.

Supplies

Most facilities use plastic preheparinized syringe/needle assemblies for arterial collection. According to the Clinical and Laboratory Standards Institute, vacuum tubes, which contain subatmospheric pressure, should not be used to collect blood gas specimens (4). Additionally, the heparin in heparinized specimen collection tubes may not be suitable for the specific arterial analytes to be tested or the method of analysis. Avoid using needles larger than 22 gauge, which may be too big to access the radial artery. A 23-gauge needle is optimum. Prepare the needle and syringe according to manufacturer's recommendations. The use of a tourniquet is not necessary.

Procedure

Arterial access procedures require the same considerations as venipuncture procedures in regards to the following:

- Standard precautions
- Patient identification

- Introduction and statement of purpose to the patient
- Positioning the patient for stability and safety
- Site preparation
- Warning the patient of the imminent puncture
- Removing the needle if the patient experiences excruciating pain
- Bandaging the patient after stasis is complete
- Labeling specimens at the patient's side
- Recording specimen collection information

Patients subjected to arterial blood gas analysis should be in a resting or "steady state" for at least 20 minutes prior to specimen collection in order to obtain meaningful data. Changes to one's respiratory status (i.e., changes to ventilator settings or oxygen therapy) should be constant for at least 20 minutes prior to collection.

Radial Artery

Prior to performing a radial artery puncture, establish that adequate collateral circulation exists so that blood will continue to feed the hand should the radial puncture result in damage to the artery. The presence of collateral circulation is determined by performing the modified Allen test (Box 5.1). If positive, prepare the site for arterial access by cleansing the skin above the radial artery with the appropriate antiseptic according to facility policy.

If possible, hyperextend the patient's hand to bring the artery close to the surface of the skin, to firmly anchor the artery, and to stretch the skin for ease of needle insertion. If the patient is not conscious and cannot comply, facilitate hyperextension by placing a rolled towel under the lower forearm. Position the index finger of your free hand on the skin directly over the artery with gentle pressure so the artery can be located by its pulse, but not enough pressure to constrict blood flow. Hold the syringe in your dominant hand between the thumb and index finger, like a dart. Warn the patient of

---

BOX 5.1   Modified Allen Test

Step 1. Instruct the patient to clench his/her fist.

Step 2. Constrict the radial and ulnar arteries by applying bilateral pressure.

Step 3. Instruct the patient to open his/her fist. The palm should be pale in color indicating circulation to the hand has been occluded.

Step 4. Release pressure to the ulnar artery while maintaining pressure to the radial artery.

Step 5. Observe for the return of normal skin tone to the hand (a positive Allen test), indicating circulation has been restored. If positive, proceed with the radial puncture. If negative (palm remains in pallor), seek an alternative site.

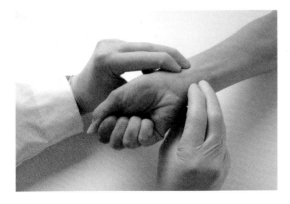

FIGURE 5.12 The presence of collateral circulation is determined by performing the modified Allen test.

the imminent puncture and insert the needle at a low angle (less than 45 degrees) with the bevel up and with a steady advance, slightly distal to your finger. (See Figs. 5.12 to 5.18.)

 According to the Standards . . . arterial blood for blood gas analysis should not be drawn into vacuum tubes, which contain subatmospheric pressure.

Brachial Artery

Position the patient's arm on a firm surface (e.g., inpatient: on the bed or bedside table; outpatient: on the arm rest of a phlebotomy chair). Prepare the site with the appropriate antiseptic according to facility policy. Place the index finger and second finger of your free hand on the skin directly over the artery with space between for needle insertion. Apply gentle pressure so that the artery can be located by its pulse, but not enough pressure to constrict blood flow. Hold the syringe in your dominant hand between the thumb and index finger, like a dart, at an angle less than 45 degrees with the bevel up. Warn the patient of the imminent puncture and insert the needle with a steady advance.

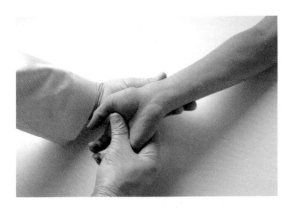

FIGURE 5.13 Hyperextend the patient's wrist if possible to bring the artery closer to the surface of the skin.

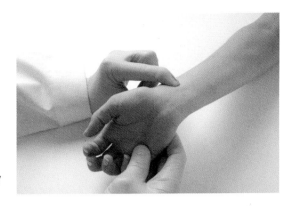

FIGURE 5.14 Locate the artery by feeling for a pulse.

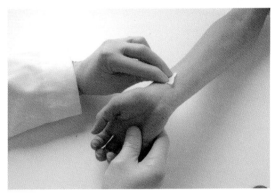

FIGURE 5.15 Cleanse the site.

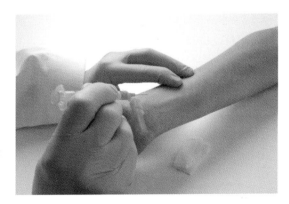

FIGURE 5.16 Insert the needle at a 45-degree angle or less and allow the syringe to fill until the appropriate quantity is obtained.

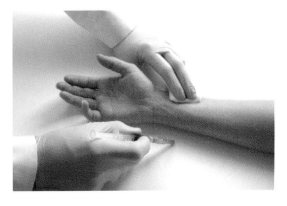

FIGURE 5.17 Remove the needle and conceal the contaminated sharp immediately.

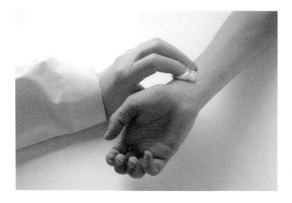

FIGURE 5.18 Hold pressure. Apply at least 5 minutes of pressure.

Completing the Procedure

When the artery is accessed, blood should flow into the syringe without assistance. Allow the syringe to fill until an adequate volume has been obtained according to the requirements of the testing facility. Place a gauze pad lightly over the insertion point, remove the needle quickly, and then apply firm pressure for 3 to 5 minutes. Immediately activate the needle's safety feature or imbed the tip of the needle into the concealment material (e.g., rubber or plastic block) provided by the manufacturer. This preserves the concentration of gases in the sample and provides a temporary means of concealment of the contaminated sharp. Invert or roll the syringe to fully mix with the anticoagulant and expel any trapped air bubbles according to manufacturer's recommendations. Record information pertinent to the patient's respiratory therapy on the test request form (e.g., ventilator settings, oxygen therapy, etc.). Bandage the puncture site after ensuring that bleeding has stopped from both the artery and the surface of the skin. This is best accomplished by observing the site for several seconds for superficial bleeding and hematoma formation. If bleeding continues, apply additional pressure until stasis is complete. Then bandage the site with a pressure bandage. Observe the skin below the puncture site for normal coloration and temperature. Notify the patient's physician or immediate caregiver if hemostasis is prolonged or if the skin below the puncture indicates impaired circulation.

Complications

Missed Artery

If the radial artery is missed, slowly withdraw the needle until the bevel is barely beneath the surface of the skin. If flow does not begin, repalpate for the location of the artery, move the needle in the appropriate direction, and advance it without probing. Probing for an artery that cannot be palpated in an attempt to blindly access it risks injury to the patient and subjects the facility to liability. If a calculated relocation cannot be performed with confidence that the artery can be accessed safely or successfully, remove the needle, apply firm pressure, and repeat the procedure on another site.

Needle relocation should not be considered to recover a failed attempt to access the brachial artery (Fig. 5.19). The close proximity of the median nerves makes needle relocation risky and subjects the patient to an increased potential for injury.

Nerve Involvement

If at any time the patient expresses excruciating pain, an electriclike or shooting pain sensation, or tingling or numbness in the fingers, remove the needle immediately and apply pressure. These symptoms indicate the needle has come in contact with a nerve. Any movement of the needle can result in further or permanent injury. Treat the patient according to the severity of the symptoms as directed by facility policy. Record the specifics of the incident with attention to detail according to your facility's incident reporting protocol.

Hematoma

Nerves can also be injured by the pressure applied to them from hematomas. Due to the increased pressure in arteries, hematoma formation is more likely during or after arterial punctures than venipunctures. Healthcare personnel drawing arterial specimens must be aware of this increased potential and be prepared to terminate a puncture should hematoma formation occur before the procedure is complete. With the same degree of caution, those performing arterial punctures must diligently apply pressure to the site after completing the procedure. After applying 3 to 5 minutes of pressure, observe radial or brachial puncture sites for the raising or mounding of the tissue that would indicate that the puncture in the artery has not sealed. At least 5 seconds of observation are necessary before bandaging to ensure that stasis is complete.

Syncope

As stated in Chapters 3 and 7, syncope is a risk of phlebotomy. Be prepared for all patients to lose consciousness. Watch for the signs of an imminent loss of consciousness including pallor, perspiration, hyperventilation, anxiety, etc. and be prepared to react. Should the patient lose consciousness during the procedure, remove the needle immediately, apply pressure, and activate the needle's safety feature before tending to the patient. Lower the patient's head

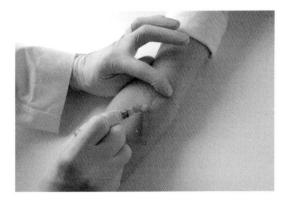

FIGURE 5.19 Needle relocation should not be considered to recover a failed attempt to access the brachial artery.

below the plane of the heart and/or apply a cold compress to the forehead or back of the neck. Assess all patients prior to leaving for the signs of vertigo (dizziness) or syncope. Allow patients demonstrating any such symptoms adequate time to recover before releasing them. If necessary, have the patient assessed by a physician. (See Chapter 3 for more information on managing patients with vertigo and syncope.)

Specimen Transport

After collecting the specimen and bandaging the patient, transport the arterial specimen to the testing facility as soon as possible. If collected in a plastic syringe and it is anticipated that testing will be completed within 30 minutes, transport the specimen at room temperature (4,8). If it is anticipated that testing will be delayed, collect the specimen into an appropriately heparinized glass syringe and transport on ice. Delays in testing specimens collected in plastic syringes can result in an increase in the measured PO_2 (9,10). If the patient is dependent on Medicare to cover the expense of oxygen therapy, an erroneously elevated PO_2 level can deprive the patient of coverage to which he/she is entitled. A more serious consequence is that the patient may not receive the therapy the body requires because of an erroneous result, further compromising his or her healthcare.

BLOOD CULTURE COLLECTION

An improperly collected blood culture can impact the patient unlike any other collection error. When bacteria enter a blood culture vial from sources external to the patient, the patient can be treated as if he or she has a bacterial infection. Treatment for a false-positive blood culture has been shown to increase a patient's hospital stay by 4.5 days and add more than $5,000 to the cost of treatment (adjusted for inflation since the study was published) (11,12). More importantly, it can keep patients from rejoining their families and jobs and reclaiming their daily lives. Conversely, improper blood culture collection errors can yield negative results in patients who actually have bacteria in their blood stream leading to life-threatening delays in treatment and, potentially, death.

Bacteria frequently enter the blood stream in many ways without adversely affecting individuals with healthy immune systems. Breaks in the skin, dental procedures, mucous membranes, and other routes of entry into the blood provide ready access to potentially infectious microorganisms. In the healthy individual, the body's cellular and immune responses engulf invading organisms before they are able to multiply. However, if the patient is acutely ill and/or immunocompromised, bacteria can develop into a potentially fatal systemic infection (septicemia). Early detection and treatment depends upon collecting blood cultures properly. Healthcare personnel who are not aware of the important aspects of blood culture collection can commit errors that cause rampant bacterial infections to go undetected and untreated (false-negative). Likewise, poor technique can cause patients to be treated for bacterial infections they don't have (false-positive). (See "In the Lab," later in this chapter.)

Preventing False-Negatives

Some bacteria, such as *Escherichia coli*, can exist in the blood stream in quantities as low as 1 organism per milliliter of blood. To recover such low-titer organisms, it is necessary to withdraw large volumes of blood from separate venipunctures. For adult patients, the optimal volume for each set of blood cultures is 20 to 30 mL of blood per set distributed between two bottles (13). For infants and children, 1 to 5 mL per set is preferred unless the patient's body weight indicates smaller volumes. (See Table 4.1, Chapter 4.) These lesser volumes require inoculation into pediatric blood culture vials to ensure the proper blood:broth dilution is maintained (between 1:5 and 1:10). When healthcare personnel collect less than these recommended volumes, the potential to recover the causative organism is compromised and risks a delay in detection and treatment.

 Tips from the Trenches: When healthcare personnel collect inadequate volumes of blood for blood cultures, it puts the patient at risk of a potentially fatal delay in detection and treatment.

To facilitate the recovery of microorganisms that can exist in low quantities, physicians usually order several sets of blood cultures collected at different times and/or from different sites. One set of blood cultures consists of two bottles inoculated with blood drawn from the same venipuncture (Fig. 5.20) (13). Multiple sets are never to be drawn and inoculated with the blood drawn from one venipuncture. If multiple sets are ordered, they may be

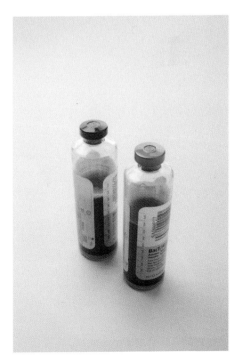

FIGURE 5.20 One set of blood cultures is defined as two bottles inoculated with blood drawn from one venipuncture.

collected at the same time in two consecutive venipunctures in different sites or from the same site at intervals of 15 to 45 minutes. The reason for performing separate venipunctures for each set is that if the site was not properly disinfected or if the collector failed to exercise aseptic technique, all bottles filled from the same draw are likely to be falsely positive. In contrast, when drawn separately, poor technique is less likely to result in the contamination of both sets.

 Tips from the Trenches: *Healthcare personnel should avoid the temptation to draw two sets of blood cultures from one venipuncture for expediency. By definition, multiple bottles filled from a single venipuncture constitute a single blood culture (13).*

Preventing False-Positives

One study reports that average hospital charges for patients with false-positive blood cultures is more than 50% higher than for similar patients with true-negative cultures (14). Bacteria from outside the patient's blood stream can contaminate blood culture bottles during the collection process in many ways (Fig. 5.21):

- When puncture sites are not prepared aseptically
- When the decontamination solution has not been allowed adequate time to kill surface bacteria
- When friction to expose underlying bacteria to the antiseptic is insufficient
- When equipment is contaminated during use
- When the tops of blood culture bottles are contaminated
- When puncture sites are recontaminated by palpation after initial cleansing

Careful attention to the finer points of blood culture collection is critical for blood culture results to reflect the patient's actual status. Blood cultures contaminated during the collection process have been shown to increase

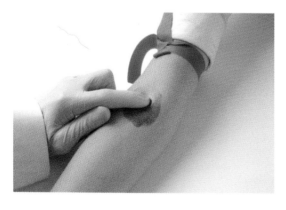

FIGURE 5.21 Bacteria from outside the patient's blood stream can contaminate the collection in many ways.

microbiology department expenditures towards overtime hours by at least 30% (3). In one study, 26% of all pediatric outpatients collected for blood cultures were subsequently hospitalized as a result of a contaminated blood culture (15).

Several strategies have been identified to be effective in reducing the frequency of false-positive blood cultures:

- Use of a designated blood culture collection team
- Use of commercial prep kits
- Use of tincture of iodine instead of iodophors
- Use of "collector feedback" technique

Designated Blood Culture Collection Team

A study released by the College of American Pathologists (CAP) in 1998, showed several key elements contribute to high contamination rates (16). One of them involves the personnel designated to collect blood cultures. Blood cultures collected by personnel who were not members of a team designated specifically for blood collection had a significantly higher contamination rate (77%) than those drawn by members of a designated phlebotomy team. In fact, the lowest contamination rate was associated with facilities in which 90% or more of the blood cultures were collected by a designated phlebotomy staff. A second study found a dramatic reduction in blood culture contamination (up to 86%) when a trained blood culture collection team was instituted (Table 5.2) (14).

Several studies project the overall cost savings to a facility when a dedicated phlebotomy team is employed to collect blood cultures (14,16,17). One study calculates that the savings associated with using a phlebotomy service to be $20 per blood culture specimen collected (17). Another report projected that the 487-bed facility studied might save as much as $1.2 million annually if it employed a dedicated phlebotomy team to collect blood cultures (14).

Unfortunately, many facilities no longer have the luxury of maintaining a team of phlebotomists. For these facilities it is critically important to continuously educate and monitor those collecting blood cultures to prevent unnecessary stays and their associated costs.

TABLE 5.2 ▪ Contamination Rates of Blood Cultures Drawn By Phlebotomy Team Versus Nonphlebotomy Team		
	Facilities in Which Most Cultures Were Drawn By a Team of Phlebotomists	**Facilities in Which Most Cultures Were Drawn By Nonphlebotomists**
Weinbaum et al. (Unit A)[14]	1.2	8.4
Wienbaum et al. (Unit B)[14]	1.0	4.8
Schifman et al.[16]	2.2	3.9

Commercial Skin Prep Kits

Although separately packaged alcohol preps and povidone swabs are available for site preparation, studies show that they are less effective than the commercially prepared prep kits (18). Such kits increase the cost per collection, but compared to the cost of a high contamination rate, converting to commercially prepared prep kits can lower the overall costs considerably (Fig. 5.22). A number of kits are available including the Cepti-Seal and ChloraPrep (Mediflex Hospital Products, Overland Park, KS, USA) and Persist (BD, Franklin Lakes, NJ, USA).

Disinfectants

Until recently, iodine-based antiseptics (sometimes used in conjunction with isopropyl alcohol) have been the industry standard for sterilizing puncture sites prior to blood culture collection. Facilities using iodine as a disinfectant for blood culture site preparation should know that puncture sites prepared using iodine tincture as opposed to an iodophor (e.g., povidone) have been found to be superior in combating contamination at sites where nonphlebotomy personnel collect cultures (16). A second study showed that iodine tincture is more effective than an iodophor where cultures are not collected by a designated phlebotomy team (19).

However, iodine readily absorbs into the skin and is toxic to the liver and thyroid. In addition, some patients have iodine sensitivity. For these reasons, chlorhexidine has gradually emerged as the preferred skin disinfectant in many applications. Studies find it to be more effective than povidone iodine in skin asepsis (20). It has also been reported that chlorhexidine demonstrates a low incidence of hypersensitivity and skin irritation and that there is no evidence of toxicity (21).

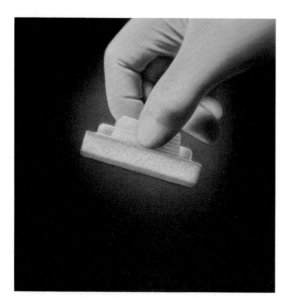

FIGURE 5.22 Chloraprep (courtesy of MediFlex). Studies show that commercially prepared blood culture prep kits are more effective than separately packaged alcohol preps and povidone swabs.

Collector Feedback

One unique approach to reducing blood culture contamination rates is taking a micromanagement approach known as collector feedback. One study showed that a marked reduction in contaminated blood cultures occurred when collectors were monitored and informed of their individual contamination rates (22). This mechanism involves diligent recordkeeping, but the reduction in contamination rates makes it a cost-effective strategy.

Because of transient bacteremias and other variables, it is difficult for facilities to eliminate all clinically insignificant or erroneously positive blood cultures. However, when a facility's blood culture contamination rate exceeds 3%, it is likely that collection personnel are not collecting blood cultures with adequate attention to antiseptic technique (14). Conducting in-services on site preparation is an effective means of reducing contamination rates to acceptable levels.

Site Preparation Procedure

The single most effective means to prevent blood culture contamination is to prepare the site properly. When not aseptically prepared, the presence of normal skin flora can contaminate the blood culture bottles and compromise the physician's ability to properly manage the patient.

Step 1 ■ Release the tourniquet.

After locating the vein to be accessed, release the tourniquet. Constriction of circulation must not continue during the site preparation process because proper disinfection takes more than 1 minute, after which hemoconcentration can affect test results. (See Chapter 3.)

Step 2 ■ Conduct a friction scrub.

Because bacteria can exist below several layers of dead skin cells, proper site preparation must include a 30- to 60-second friction scrub prior to or in conjunction with the application of an effective antiseptic solution (Fig. 5.23). For all commercially prepared site preparation kits, it is important to follow manufacturer's instructions for use.

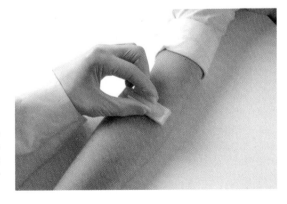

FIGURE 5.23 Proper site preparation must include a 30- to 60-second friction scrub to reach bacteria that can exist below several layers of dead skin cells.

If a commercial skin prep kit is not used, cleanse the intended puncture site initially with isopropyl alcohol and friction to remove excess surface bacteria followed by a minimum 30-second friction scrub with the disinfectant. Until recently, it has been recommended that the process is completed by placing the swab or pledget at the intended point of insertion and moving it outward in circles of increasing diameter. However, that technique is now seen as less critical than performing a diligent friction scrub and ensuring that the minimum contact time of the antiseptic with the skin is met. Allow the site to dry.

Step 3 ■ Allow the disinfectant to take effect.

Contrary to popular belief, antiseptic solutions don't kill bacteria on contact, but require at least 30 seconds of contact with the skin to become effective. Allowing the solution to dry usually provides for the minimum 30-second contact necessary to kill surface bacteria.

The bactericidal effect of iodine is directly proportional to the length of time it is allowed to remain in contact with the skin.

Some facilities instruct the collector to remove the iodine with alcohol prior to performing the puncture to prevent:

1. Absorption of iodine into the skin
2. Iodine toxicity
3. Iodine sensitivity
4. Contamination of the specimen by iodine, which can falsely increase levels of phosphorus, potassium, and uric acid (23)

Specimen Collection Procedure

While selecting and assembling the appropriate supplies and equipment for the collection, cleanse the stoppers of the blood culture bottles if recommended by the manufacturer. Although the stoppers of most blood culture bottles manufactured today are shipped sterile and protected by a protective covering, some manufacturers recommend a precautionary cleansing of the stopper with alcohol.

After the site has been cleansed and the equipment selected and assembled, retighten the tourniquet, and relocate the vein. Avoid touching the cleansed site where the needle will be inserted as this reintroduces bacteria onto the skin and potentially contaminates the collection. It is acceptable to palpate with a gloved finger above and below the intended insertion site, but once the site has been cleansed, it should not be touched prior to needle insertion. The practice of cleansing the tip of a gloved finger with the antiseptic often is mistakenly believed to be acceptable. However, unless the collector uses the same scrupulous technique to cleanse the gloved fingertip as was used to cleanse the site, including a minimum 30-second contact time with the antiseptic, the practice risks contamination of the collection and false-positive results. Perform the puncture as detailed in Chapter 3 (see Box 5.2).

Syringe Draws

Fill the syringe with enough blood to accommodate both bottles as well as any additional tests that might be ordered. When enough blood has been withdrawn (10–12 cc/bottle), terminate the venipuncture, remove the needle from the patient, and activate the safety feature of the needle. Remove the concealed sharp, replace it with a safety transfer device, and pierce the stopper of the first blood culture bottle. If the set includes aerobic and anaerobic bottles, fill the anaerobic bottle first. If the syringe is in a vertical position, air can exist at the interface of the blood and the plunger. Should the syringe be completely evacuated into the second bottle filled, any air that is pulled into an anaerobic bottle can compromise the bottle's environment enough to prevent anaerobic organisms from being detected (Box 5.2).

Once the recommended volume has been evacuated into the first blood culture bottle, evacuate the appropriate volume into the second bottle. Fill all other blood collection tubes according to the prescribed order of draw (see Chapter 3). If blood collection tubes are collected before blood culture bottles are filled, any bacteria that exist on the caps of standard blood collection tubes could be introduced into the blood culture bottles resulting in a contaminated culture. Label the specimens appropriately, bandage the site, and transport the specimens to the testing facility.

BOX 5.2   Precautionary Notes for Collecting Blood Cultures

- Do not shift your attention from the bottles while filling. If the bottles are being filled directly from a syringe, the vacuum within the bottle may pull the entire sample into the first bottle causing false-positive results from excessive white blood cells. If using a winged blood collection set, the excess vacuum in the bottle can pull more than the recommended volume of blood into the bottle. (See "In the Lab: How Blood Cultures Are Processed," this chapter.)
- Use a safety transfer device to transfer the blood from a syringe. After removing the needle from the patient, activate the safety feature, remove and discard the needle, and apply a safety transfer device that pierces the stoppers of the blood culture bottles safely.
- Do not forcefully eject the specimen from the syringe. If the blood does not evacuate from the syringe, replace the safety transfer device. Applying any force to the plunger of the syringe risks exposure from blood splatter.
- Ensure that air does not enter anaerobic bottles while filling. After filling, syringes may have an air bubble that can compromise an anaerobic environment. Should it be expelled into an anaerobic bottle, it can prevent anaerobic bacteria from multiplying and lead to false-negative results.
- When filling blood culture vials through a winged blood collection set, do not fill an anaerobic bottle first. The air in the tubing of the set will compromise the anaerobic environment and can prevent the growth of anaerobic organisms. Make sure an aerobic bottle is the first bottle filled when drawing through winged blood collection sets.

Vacuum-Assisted Draws

For a vacuum-assisted draw, use a winged blood collection set threaded into a tube holder appropriate for the blood collection bottle. Unless recommended by the manufacturer, bottles should never be filled through standard tube holders attached directly to the needle as one would fill other blood collection tubes because of the potential for the contents of the inverted bottle to reflux into the vein. (Currently, only blood collection bottles marketed by Trek [Westlake, OH, USA] are approved for direct filling in this manner.)

A winged blood collection set should never be used without a tube holder adapter (Fig. 5.24). If the blood culture bottle in use does not accommodate tube holders on hand, obtain the appropriate size tube holder from the manufacturer of the blood culture bottles.

When the vein is accessed, push the tube holder over the top of the aerobic blood culture bottle first, allowing the inner needle to puncture the stopper. If an anaerobic bottle is included in the set, it is important that it is not the first bottle filled. Air in the line of the winged blood collection set will compromise the anaerobic environment and limit the detection and identification of anaerobic organisms.

Allow the vacuum in the bottle to pull the specimen into the bottle to the appropriate volume; repeat for the second bottle, being careful not to overfill (Box 5.3). Tubes to be collected for additional lab work should be filled after the blood culture bottles. (See "Order of Draw," Chapter 3.) Label the specimens appropriately, bandage the site, and transport the specimens to the testing facility.

Draws Through Vascular Access Devices

Draws from vascular access devices such as arterial lines and central venous catheters are associated with high blood culture contamination rates (24–26). Because these ports pass through the skin and remain for long periods of time, they are susceptible to bacterial "colonization." Once colonized around the port, bacteria easily contaminate blood specimens withdrawn through them and inoculated into blood culture bottles. To confirm a culture is positive because of colonization in the line, a second blood culture must be drawn by venipuncture, and the results compared (27). A negative culture by venipuncture in conjunc-

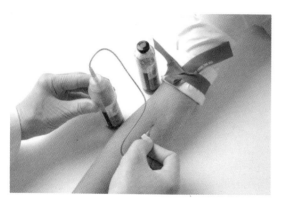

FIGURE 5.24 A winged blood collection set should never be used without a tube holder adapter.

BOX 5.3   Monitoring Fill Volumes

It is critical that blood culture bottles be filled to the volume recommended by the manufacturer, typically 10 to 12 cc per bottle for adults and 2 to 3 cc per pediatric bottle. While collection tubes for other purposes contain a vacuum calibrated to provide an optimal blood:additive ratio, blood culture bottles will fill beyond the optimum volume if filling is not monitored during collection. Since overfilling can lead to false-positive results, collectors should carefully monitor fill volumes during collection. One method is to make a mark on the bottle's label to indicate the level at which an appropriate volume of blood will have been added. (Manufacturers print volume gradations on the label to assist in establishing proper fill volumes.) Once the mark is made, collectors can simply allow the vacuum to pull blood into the broth until the level in the bottle reaches the mark.

---

tion with a positive culture by line draw confirms colonization, whereas positive cultures drawn from both sites confirm bacteremia. However, if the venipuncture culture was contaminated during collection by poor technique, the physician can be misled into concluding that the patient has a systemic bacterial infection when he/she does not. The identification of different organisms can prove the venipuncture specimen was contaminated during the collection, but the uncertainty of positive results from different sites can lead to unnecessary treatment and an extended length of stay.

Because drawing blood cultures from vascular access devices often results in contamination and require confirmatory venipunctures that consume valuable hospital resources, they should be avoided whenever possible (25) (Fig. 5.25).

IN THE LAB

How Blood Cultures Are Processed

When a blood culture set arrives in the laboratory, testing personnel typically process the specimen by immediately checking for the presence of bacteria. A

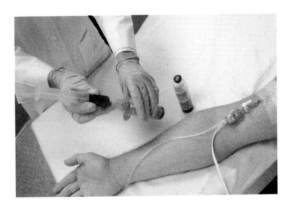

FIGURE 5.25 Because drawing blood cultures from vascular access devices often results in contamination, they should be avoided whenever possible.

drop of the inoculated broth is aspirated from the bottle, placed on a slide, and allowed to dry. The tech then performs a Gram's stain and looks for organisms under a microscope. If bacteria are seen, the physician is notified immediately. Regardless of the results of the Gram's stain, all bottles are incubated for at least 5 days (or up to 6 weeks for fungal cultures) and checked periodically during incubation for bacterial growth. Testing personnel in laboratories without blood culture instrumentation manually inoculate a sample of the broth periodically onto solid culture media (agar) that facilitates bacterial growth. When growth is visibly detected on the media, a Gram's stain is performed and the physician is notified of the results.

However, in most large hospitals and laboratories an automated blood culture incubator monitors carbon dioxide levels within the bottle, some as often as every 10 minutes. As bacteria multiply, the concentration of carbon dioxide increases within the bottle. When automated systems detect a change in the CO_2 concentration, testing personnel are alerted and another Gram's stain is performed on a drop of the bottle's contents. If bacteria are detected under microscopy, the physician is notified.

Carbon dioxide is also produced by white blood cells (WBCs), but in quantities that are usually too minuscule to trigger automated systems. However, should a blood culture bottle be overfilled, the excess WBCs can produce enough CO_2 to trigger the incubator's alarm and force unnecessary confirmatory testing. Monitoring fill volumes carefully during the collection process is the only way to prevent the unnecessary testing that is required when automated systems detect increases in CO_2 levels from nonbacterial sources.

Some blood culture systems are so sensitive that one individual microbe can multiply during incubation to detectable levels. If that microbe came from the skin because of improper site sterilization, it consumes laboratory resources unnecessarily and results in increases in laboratory and hospital costs. Because of the cost of contaminated blood cultures to the laboratory and, subsequently, the facility, it is extremely important that healthcare professionals be mindful of proper site sterilization.

REFERENCES

1. Tiosejo L, Agorrilla J. Results of blood culture contamination study in the emergency room. *Am J Infect Control* 1998;26:170.
2. Matthews D. Comparative studies of time requirement and repeat sticks during heelstick. *Neonatal Int Care* 1992;5:66–67.
3. Franck L, Gilbert R. Reducing pain during blood sampling in infants. *Clin Evid* 2002;7:352–366.
4. NCCLS. *Procedures for the collection of arterial blood specimens.* Approved Standard. H11-A3. Wayne, PA, 1999.
5. Lund C, Osborne J, Kuller J, et al. Neonatal skin care: clinical outcomes of the AWHONN/NANN Evidence-based Clinical Practice Guideline. *JOGNN* 2001;30:41–51.
6. Garza D, Becan-McBride K. *Phlebotomy handbook,* 6th ed. Upper Saddle River, NJ: Prentice Hall, 2002.
7. NCCLS. *Procedures for the collection of diagnostic blood specimens by venipuncture.* Approved Standard. H3-A5. Wayne, PA, 2003.

8. Baer, D. Blood gas specimen transport. In Zacharia M, ed. *Tips on specimen collection.* Montvale, NJ: Medical Economics, 1997:22–23.
9. Zacharia M, ed. *Tips on specimen collection.* Montvale, NJ: Medical Economics, 1997.
10. Mahoney J, Harvey J, Wong R, et al. Changes in oxygen measurements when whole blood is stored in iced plastic or glass syringes. *Clin Chem* 1991;37:1244–1248.
11. Bates DW, Goldman L, Lee TH. Contaminant blood cultures and resource utilization: the true consequences of false-positive results. *JAMA* 1991;265:365–369.
12. Schifman R. Phlebotomists at risk [Editorial]. *Mayo Clin Proc* 1998;73:703–704.
13. Dunne M, Nolte F, Wilson M. *Blood cultures III.* Cumitech 1B. Washington, D.C.: ASM Press, 1997.
14. Weinbaum FI, Lavie S, Danek M, et al. Doing it right the first time. Quality improvement and the contaminant blood culture. *J Clin Micro* 1997;35:563–565.
15. Thuler L, Jenicek M. Turegon J, et al. Impact of a false positive blood culture result on the management of febrile children. *Pediatr Infect Dis J* 1997;16:846–851.
16. Schifman R, Strand C, Meier L, et al. Blood culture contamination. *Arch Pathol Lab Med* 1998;122:216–220.
17. Schifman R. Editorial. *Mayo Clin Proc* 1998;73:703–704.
18. Schifman R, Pindur A. The effect of skin disinfection material on reducing blood culture contamination. *Am J Clin Pathol* 1993;99:536–538.
19. Strand C, Wajsbort R, Sturman K. Effect of iodophor vs tincture skin preparation on blood culture contamination rate. *JAMA* 1993;269:1004–1006.
20. Mimoz O, Karim A, Mercan A, et al. Chlorhexidine compared with povidone-iodine as skin preparation before blood culture: a randomized, controlled trial. *Ann Intern Med* 1999;131:834–837.
21. Widmere A, Frei R. *Manual of clinical microbiology,* 7th ed. Washington, DC: ASM Press, 1999:154.
22. Gibb P, Hill B, Chorel B, et al. Reduction in blood culture contamination rate by feedback to phlebotomists. *Arch Pathol Lab Med* 1997;121:503–507.
23. Becan-McBride, K (ed). Preanalytical phase and important requisite of laboratory testing. *Adv Med Lab Prof* 1998;Sept:12–17.
24. Garza D, Becan-McBride K. *Phlebotomy handbook,* 5th ed. Upper Saddle River, NJ: Prentice Hall; 1999.
25. Norberg A, Christopher N, Ramundo M, et al. Contamination rates of blood cultures obtained by dedicated phlebotomy vs intravenous catheter. *JAMA.*2003;289:726–729.
26. Levin P, Hersch M, Rudensky B, et al. The use of the arterial line as a source for blood cultures. *Intens Care Med* 2000;26:1350–1354.
27. Beutz M, Sherman G, Mayfield J, et al. Clinical utility of blood cultures drawn from central vein catheters and peripheral venipuncture in critically ill medical patients. *Chest* 2003;123:854–861.

REVIEW QUESTIONS

1. The concentrations of which of the following analytes differs in venous versus arterial specimens?
    a. ammonia
    b. creatinine
    c. phosphorus
    d. hemoglobin
2. Which site is acceptable for an arterial blood gas puncture?
    a. the median artery
    b. the basilic artery
    c. the brachial artery
    d. the carotid artery
3. Which artery is the preferred artery for performing an arterial puncture?
    a. the femoral artery
    b. the ulnar artery
    c. the brachial artery
    d. the radial artery
4. The brachial artery should be considered only if:
    a. requested by the physician
    b. it has been determined neither radial artery can be safely and successfully accessed
    c. the femoral artery is not accessible
    d. the patient is on a respirator
5. Changes to ventilator settings or oxygen therapy should be constant for at least _____ minutes prior to collection.
    a. 10
    b. 20
    c. 30
    d. 60
6. The modified Allen test determines:
    a. the presence of collateral circulation to the hand
    b. the patient's clotting ability
    c. false-positive blood cultures
    d. oxygen saturation
7. Use of a multiskilled workforce to draw blood specimens:
    a. increases blood culture contamination rates
    b. minimizes the number of collection errors
    c. results in substantial overall cost savings
    d. dramatically reduces detection of transient bacteremia
8. The single most important factor in collecting uncontaminated blood cultures is:
    a. highly dedicated personnel
    b. proper collection site preparation
    c. use of winged infusion (butterfly) devices
    d. changing the needle on the syringe before evacuating specimen into culture bottle

9. The American Society for Microbiology standards call for a rate of blood culture contamination that does not exceed:
   a. 1%
   b. 2%
   c. 3%
   d. 5%
10. Chlorhexidine has been found to be more effective than _____ in decontaminating sites for blood culture collection.
    a. alcohol
    b. povidone iodine compounds
    c. Hibiclens
    d. bactericidal soaps
11. If filling both aerobic and anaerobic vials with a syringe:
    a. inoculate the aerobic vial first so that any air in the syringe doesn't compromise the aerobic environment
    b. inoculate the anaerobic vial first so that any air in the syringe doesn't compromise the anaerobic environment
    c. inoculate the aerobic vial first to prevent additive carryover
    d. hold the vials in one hand while piercing the stopper with the syringe in the other.
12. Contaminated blood cultures have been found to:
    a. be a result of nosocomial infections
    b. increase a patient's length of stay up to 4 days and add more than $4,000 to the cost of treatment
    c. increase a patient's length of stay up to 4.5 days and add more than $5,000 to the cost of treatment
    d. increase the cost of overtime expenditures in the phlebotomy department due to recollection.
13. When collecting capillary blood from a newborn:
    a. never prewarm the heel
    b. perform the puncture on the medial or lateral aspect of the heel
    c. make two punctures in the center of the heel
    d. a crib card constitutes positive identification
14. Compared to venous blood, capillary specimens have significantly higher concentrations of:
    a. glucose
    b. potassium
    c. total protein
    d. calcium
15. When prewarming the site of a skin puncture, the temperature of the warming device should not exceed:
    a. 25°C
    b. 30°C
    c. 35°C
    d. 42°C

Specimen Handling, Storage, and Transportation

6

KEY TERMS AND DEFINITIONS

Analytes Components of blood that are tested by a clinical laboratory.

Plasma The liquid portion of the blood after centrifugation of a specimen in which an anticoagulant has prevented clot formation.

Preanalytical errors Those errors that affect a test result from the time a test is ordered until the specimen is tested.

Serum The liquid portion of the blood after centrifugation of a specimen that is allowed to clot (red top tubes).

Whole blood Blood in which coagulation is inhibited by the activity of anticoagulants and the cellular material is allowed to remain in suspension with the plasma. Uncentrifuged anticoagulated blood.

Note: The list of handling, storage, and transportation requirements for every lab test is extensive and beyond the scope of this text. The information presented here is intended to provide general handling, storage, and transportation guidelines for blood specimens to be tested in a clinical laboratory. Because there are no rules of specimen transportation and storage that can be universally applied to all tubes for all tests all of the time, those collecting blood specimens should consult their testing laboratory for any specific requirements relating to the analyte to be tested.

INTRODUCTION

Although specimen collection is critical, the influence the blood collector has on results doesn't end when the blood fills the tube. Disregarding errors that can occur during specimen handling, storage, and transport can significantly alter test results. If healthcare professionals don't recognize and avoid processing errors, inaccurate results can be reported and impact a patient's diagnosis, medication, treatment, and general management with life-threatening consequences.

This chapter discusses the handling of blood after collection to minimize the erroneous results processing errors can produce. Upon completing this chapter, the reader should be able to:

- Identify errors in specimen transportation and processing that can significantly alter results
- List the analytes affected by delayed processing
- Discuss the effects time, temperature, and storage conditions can have on test results
- Apply highly referenced information on specimen collection errors to reduce the introduction of preanalytical errors into the specimens that are transported and/or processed

GENERAL CONSIDERATIONS

From the moment the blood enters the tube, significant and irreversible changes begin to take place. Proper specimen handling assures the result reported reflects the concentration in which the analyte exists in the patient as precisely as technologically possible.

Once outside of the circulatory system, blood is subject to the effects of time, temperature, light, and other natural processes that take place when blood is no longer in circulation (Fig. 6.1). The race against the effects of these processes begins the moment blood enters the collection tube and continues until the specimen is analyzed. Those factors that alter test results include clotting, glycolysis, and the transfer of ions between serum and red blood cells. Clotting can be prevented by properly mixing tubes containing anticoagulants immediately on collection (see Chapter 3). Minimizing glycolysis and ion exchange, however, requires proper handling throughout the preanalytical phase of clinical testing.

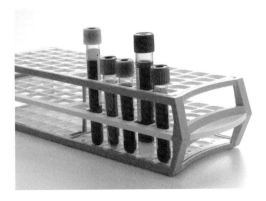

FIGURE 6.1 Once outside of the circulatory system, blood is subject to the effects of time, temperature, light, and other natural processes that take place when blood is no longer in circulation.

Tips from the Trenches: *Healthcare personnel who disregard the effects that time, temperature, and light have on blood specimens can introduce preanalytical errors into the specimen that dramatically alter results, leading to patient mismanagement and medical errors.*

Preventing Glycolysis and Ion Exchange

Glycolysis refers to the metabolism of glucose. When serum or plasma remains in contact with red blood cells during specimen transport and storage, glycolysis can result in falsely lower glucose results. At its peak, glycolysis can decrease the concentration of glucose in the serum or plasma at the rate of up to 200 mg/L per hour (1). This process accelerates at higher temperatures and with elevated white blood cell counts. When specimens cannot be immediately centrifuged and the serum or plasma separated from the cells (e.g., specimens drawn in patients' homes or long-term care facilities where there is no access to processing equipment), glucose levels can be preserved two ways: (1) by collecting the specimen into tubes containing sodium fluoride or sodium or potassium oxalate (gray stopper tubes) or (2) by refrigeration. Each has its limitations and neither provides an alternative to centrifugation and separation of the serum or plasma from the cells when other chemistry tests are drawn at the same time. For example, fluoride or oxalate preservatives are not appropriate for any other analyte. So when multiple tests have been ordered, other tubes must be collected.

Refrigeration alone is not an appropriate means of preserving specimens when tests are requested in addition to glucose. Although refrigeration inhibits glycolysis, it also promotes ion exchange because of the effect refrigeration has on a natural mechanism known as the Na^+/K^+ ATPase pump. At room temperature and higher, this pump moves sodium out of the red blood cell and moves potassium in, so much so that the concentration of potassium within the cell is 23 times greater than that of the plasma. However, at refrigerated temperatures, the pump is inhibited, allowing large quantities of K^+ ions to pour out of the cell into the serum or plasma (2). As a result, within only a few hours of contact with the cells, the potassium level can increase substantially. This can cause patients with life-threateningly low potassium levels to appear normal to the physician with potentially disastrous results. For example, if a patient with a low potassium level is drawn for tests that include potassium, any delay in processing and/or refrigeration of the specimen before centrifugation can cause potassium to leak from the cells into the serum, elevating the eventual test result reported to be within normal limits. The falsely elevated result can lead to inaction that causes complications including seizure and death. Likewise, a patient with a normal potassium level can be reported as having an abnormally high level due to delays in specimen processing or improper storage/transport conditions. This can prompt the physician to institute medical interventions that remove potassium from the body, plunging the normal patient into a life-threatening low

BOX 6.1	Analytes That Change During Serum/Cell Exposure
Increased	Decreased
Lactate dehydrogenase (LD)	Glucose
Phosphorus ($PO4^+$)	Ionized calcium (Ca^{++})
Ammonia ($NH4^-$)	Bicarbonate (CO_2)
Potassium (K^+)	Folate
Creatinine	
B-12	
ALT	
AST	

potassium state. In addition to seizure and death, both patients have the potential for other complications including:

- Cardiac arrhythmia
- Neuromuscular abnormalities
- Muscular tetany
- Respiratory arrest
- Renal dysfunction

Glucose and potassium aren't the only analytes that change in concentration when serum or plasma is exposed to red blood cells. (See Box 6.1 and Fig. 6.2.) Because of these analyte alterations, the Clinical and Laboratory Standards Institute recommends that tubes drawn for routine chemistry testing be centrifuged and separated within 2 hours of collection unless evidence exists that longer contact times do not contribute to the inaccuracy of the result (3). Therefore, if any of these analytes are scheduled for testing or if there is a potential for them to be tested during the storage of the specimen, the serum/plasma should be removed from the cells within 2 hours of collection (Fig. 6.3). This can be accomplished by collecting the specimen into a gel separator tube and centrifuging the tube within 2 hours through the use of

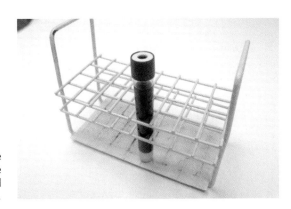

FIGURE 6.2 Many analytes are subject to change when the serum or plasma is not separated from contact with red blood cells.

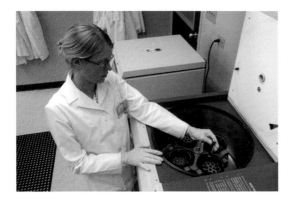

FIGURE 6.3 Tubes drawn for routine chemistry testing must be centrifuged and separated within 2 hours of collection.

other various serum separator devices or by physically removing the serum/plasma from the tube within 2 hours and transferring it to a properly labeled transfer tube.

 Tips from the Trenches: *Refrigerating clotted specimens, even for short periods of time, without separating the serum from the cells is unacceptable when testing includes potassium. Under refrigerated conditions, potassium leaks from the cells into the serum/plasma resulting in falsely elevated results.*

HANDLING

Centrifugation

Centrifugation forces all the cellular components of the blood (red cells, white cells, and platelets) to the bottom of the tube with the cell-free serum or plasma to be tested remaining above the cells. Tubes with anticoagulants can be centrifuged immediately upon collection. However, tubes without anticoagulants should be allowed to sit for 20 to 30 minutes for complete clotting to take place. This includes so-called "clot activator" tubes, which contain silica particles or other substances that facilitate complete clotting.

 Tips from the Trenches: *A common misperception is that clot-activator tubes hasten clotting and allow specimens to be centrifuged more quickly. However, the additive in such tubes facilitates complete clotting, not faster clotting. As a result, the serum from clot activator tubes is less likely to contain fibrin strands that interfere with serum recovery, but it may still take up to 30 minutes for complete clotting to occur.*

Proper centrifugation is critical. During the clotting process, platelets are activated, releasing potassium into the serum. When centrifugation is inadequate and platelets remain in the serum, the potassium level gradually increases prior to testing, significantly elevating the result to be reported and potentially leading to the same patient complications and medical errors that can occur when serum remains in contact with red blood cells. To prevent potassium contamination by platelet activation, facilities must adhere to the recommendations of the centrifuge and tube manufacturers in regard to time and relative centrifugal force (rcf). RCF, also known as g-force, can be determined by the following formula:

$$rcf = 1.11825 \times 10^{-5} \times r \times n^2$$
$$r = \text{rotating radius (cm)}$$
$$n = \text{speed of rotation (rpm)}$$

The rotating radius is described as the distance from the centrifuge's rotor axis to the bottom of the tube at its greatest horizontal distance from the rotor during centrifugation (see Appendix 6).

Because the distance from the rotor to the bottom of the tube varies from centrifuge to centrifuge, each model requires a calculation of this equation to establish the proper combination of time and speed in order to obtain the manufacturer's recommended rcf for the tube in use. For example, if the manufacturer of the tube requires an rcf of 3,000 g, and the distance from the axis of the rotor to the bottom of the tube at its greatest distance during centrifugation is 25 cm, the calculation is as follows:

$$3,000 = .0000111825 \times 25 \text{ cm} \times n^2$$

or

$$n^2 = \frac{3,000}{.0000111825 \times 25 \text{ cm}}$$

which becomes

the square root of $(\sqrt{)}10,731,053 = 3276$ rpm.

An rcf nomograph eliminates the need for this calculation (see Appendix 6).

Determining the proper combination for your facility's equipment is critical to obtaining serum potassium levels that are not altered by platelet activation. To minimize the potential for erroneous potassium results, many facilities use a heparinized (green stopper) tube for electrolyte testing in which clotting does not occur and platelets are not activated (see Fig. 6.3).

Serum Separators

To facilitate specimen processing, a wide variety of serum separators are available that separate the serum from the cells. Some collection tubes contain a gel-type serum separator, which forms a physical barrier between the cells and the serum during centrifugation, negating the need to physically remove the serum from the tube. With this barrier in place, glycolysis and ion transfer are interrupted. When stored at the proper temperature, serum or plasma can be exposed to the gel barrier for 2 to 5 days. However, once gel-

---

BOX 6.2   Recentrifuging Gel Tubes

Occasionally, additional serum than that separated from the cells upon initial centrifugation is required for testing. However, spinning gel separator tubes a second time to obtain more serum should not be conducted after 2 hours from the time of collection. If the second centrifugation is conducted after 2 hours from collection, the process ultimately combines serum/plasma that has been in contact with the cells—and undergoing dramatic changes—to the serum/plasma separated in a timely manner. The combined serum/plasma then becomes a hybrid concentration, yielding altered results for many analytes. Therefore, gel separator tubes should not be recentrifuged and used for testing any analytes affected by serum-cell contact. Testing such a specimen can result in erroneous results and patient mismanagement.

---

separator tubes have been centrifuged and stored, repeat centrifugation should not be conducted (see Box 6.2).

Some analytes are adversely affected by prolonged contact with some gel barriers. The US Food and Drug Administration (FDA) has approved the gel tubes of some manufacturers for all analytes while those of other manufacturers have been shown to affect the results of some therapeutic drugs. Therefore, it is prudent to avoid collecting any therapeutic drug tests into gel- separator tubes unless confirmed that the gel of the tube in use is inert. Table 6.1 lists some of the analytes that can be affected when stored in a gel-separator tube.

 Tips from the Trenches: Once gel-separator tubes have been centrifuged and stored, repeat centrifugation should not be conducted.

Alternatives to gel serum separators include devices added to the specimen prior to centrifugation and those that are used after centrifugation.

TABLE 6.1 ▦ Analytes Affected by Storage in Gel-Separator Tubes (3,4)	
Therapeutic Drugs*	**Other Analytes**
Phenytoin (Dilantin**)	Tricyclic antidepressants
Phenobarbital	(amitriptyline, imipramine, etc.)
Quinidine	Progesterone
Carbamazepine (Tegretol***)	Direct antiglobulin tests
Lidocaine	Ionized calcium

*Gel-separator tubes from some manufacturers are inert. Consult package inserts accompanying gel-separator tubes for brand-specific limitations.
**Dilantin is a registered trademark of Parke-Davis (Morris Plains, NJ, USA).
***Tegretol is a registered trademark of Novartis Pharmaceuticals Corp. (East Hanover, NJ, USA).

Manufacturer's recommendations on use and storage limitations should be consulted and followed to ensure specimen stability.

Some facilities use plunger-type serum separators to remove serum or plasma from the cells. These devices consist of a plastic tube with an opening at one end and a filter device on the other. After centrifugation, the stopper of the tube is removed and the device inserted, filter end first, and pressed though the serum or plasma. The liquid portion of the specimen to be tested flows through the filter and into the plastic tube facilitating separation from the cells and providing a convenient means to pour the serum or plasma into a transfer tube or testing cup.

However, caution should be exercised when storing serum or plasma in these devices for two reasons. First, the risk of splashes to the face exposes the user to the potential to acquire a bloodborne pathogen. The US Occupational Safety and Health Administration (OSHA) insists that whenever it is reasonable to expect an exposure to occur, proper protective equipment must be used. Second, unless the device is withdrawn to create an air space between the cells and the filtering unit, complete separation from the cells may not occur and irreversible changes in the specimen could take place during storage. If the device does not prevent the backflow of serum through the filter, establishing an air space may not be possible. In such cases, complete separation will require the serum or plasma to be transferred from the separator into another tube. If an air space can be created, storage and further testing should only be conducted if the device's manufacturer has appropriate documentation that storage in the device does not affect the analytes to be tested.

 According to the Standards. . . . . . An air barrier should be created between the cells and the bottom of plunger-type serum separators to prevent ion exchange through the device's filter.

Transfer Tubes

To completely remove serum or plasma from the tube into which blood was collected, some facilities pour or aspirate an aliquot into a plastic transfer tube with a screw cap or tight-fitting closure (Fig. 6.4.) This process provides the greatest assurance against the effects of cell contact and offers processing personnel a convenient way to manage specimens that require transportation to multiple testing stations or facilities. Proper personal protective equipment must be used, including an impermeable gown or lab coat, gloves, and eye protection (5). Transfer tubes must be completely labeled with the appropriate patient information to assure complete and accurate specimen identification.

 Tips from the Trenches: Proper personal protective equipment must be used including an impermeable gown or lab coat, gloves, and eye protection when physically transferring specimens from one tube to another.

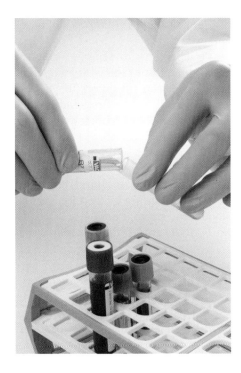

FIGURE 6.4 Some facilities pour or aspirate an aliquot of serum or plasma into a plastic transfer tube for storage or transportation.

Analytes Unstable after Separation

For many tests, separated serum or plasma is stable at room temperature up to 8 hours after collection; many analytes have longer stability. However, unless the testing facility requires separated serum/plasma to remain at room temperature, refrigerating separated specimens ensures analytes will remain stable (Table 6.2).

Some tests collected in heparinized (green top) tubes require the specimen to be immediately chilled. If these tests are ordered in addition to potassium, collect a separate tube for the potassium, keep it at room temperature, and separate the plasma from the cells within 2 hours. If there is any question, consult the testing facility for specific handling, storage, and transportation requirements with regard to the test in question.

Handling Coagulation Specimens

Sodium citrate tubes for coagulation studies can remain at room temperature after collection (6). However, it is recommended that activated partial thromboplastin times (aPTTs) be tested within 4 hours. If the patient is heparinized, specimens for aPTT testing should be centrifuged, the plasma removed from the cells within 1 hour after collection and tested within 4 hours. Protimes, however, are more forgiving; they are stable for up to 24 hours at room temperature, even uncentrifuged. When testing is delayed beyond these limitations, specimens for coagulation studies should be cen-

TABLE 6.2 ■ Analyte Stability

Analyte Stability Before Centrifugation and Separation from Cells

Analyte	Room Temperature	Refrigerated
Albumin	At least 6 hours[3]	
ALT	24 hours[3]	
AST	24 hours[3]	
Bicarbonate	6 hours[3]	7 days[7]
Bilirubin	3 days[7]	
Calcium (ionized)	2 hours[3]	
Chloride	6 hours[3]	
Creatinine	24 hours[3]	
Glucose	2 hours[3]	< 2 hours[3]
Glucose (in fluoride tube)	1 week[7]	1 week[7]
HDL cholesterol	6 hours[1,3]	
Iron	8 hours[3]	
LDH	2 hours[3]	
Magnesium (ionized)	6 hours[3]	5 days[3]
Phosphorous	3 hours[1,3]	
Potassium	2 hours[2,3]	< 2 hours[3]
Prothrombin time	24 hours[6]	7 hours[2,6]
PTT	4 hours[6]	4 hours
PTT (patient on unfractionated heparin)	1 hour[6]	1 hour[6]
Sodium	7 days[7]	1 day[3,4]
Total protein	48 hours[3]	
Tricyclic antidepressants	N/A	6 days[3]

Stability of Whole Blood Analytes

Test	Room Temperature	Refrigerated
WBC (normal or elevated counts)	3 days to 1 week[10]	1 week[7]
WBC (low counts)	<1 day[10]	1 week[7]
Automated differential	<1 day[10]	N/A
RBC	At least 1 week[7,10]	At least 1 week[7]
HGB	At least 1 week[7,10]	At least 1 week[7]
HCT	1–2 days[7,10]	5 days[7]
PLT	1 day[7] to at least 4 days[10]	At least 24 hours[7]
MCV	1–2 days[7,10]	At least 24 hours[7]
MCH	At least 1 week[10]	N/A
Sedimentation rate	4 hours[8]	12 hours[8]
RETIC	6 hours[9]	72 hours[9]

(continues)

TABLE 6.2 ■ Analyte Stability *(continued)*		
Analyte Stability after Separation from Cells[7]		
Analyte	**Room Temperature**	**Refrigerated**
ALT	1 day	3 days
Alkaline Phosphatase	4 hours	N/A
Amylase	1 week	2 months
AST	3 days	1 week
Calcium	7 days	10 days
Bilirubin	2 days	7 days
Free T4	1 week	N/A
GGT	1 month	1 month
HCG	N/A	4 days
FE/TIBC	N/A	1 week
LDH	2–3 days	N/A
TSH	N/A	4 days
T3	2 weeks	N/A
URIC	3 days	7 days

(From Center for Phlebotomy Education, Inc. 2003, with permission.)

trifuged and the plasma separated and frozen at −20°C for up to 2 weeks (−70°C for up to 6 months) in a freezer that does not have a defrost cycle that could thaw and refreeze the specimen periodically during storage. Prior to testing, frozen specimens should be thawed at 37°C with gentle agitation and tested immediately. If immediate testing is not possible, thawed specimens may be refrigerated as long as testing takes place within 2 hours.

These limitations reflect the Clinical and Laboratory Standards Institute guidelines (6). Some laboratories may have conducted studies that demonstrate longer stability. Therefore, collectors should adhere to the protocol recommended by the testing facility.

Handling Whole Blood Specimens

For complete blood counts (CBCs), EDTA tubes can remain at room temperature without affecting cell counts or morphology if testing is to be performed within 24 hours (Box 6.3). (See Table 6.2.) Some components of a CBC have been shown to be stable at room temperature for up to 1 week (10). However, automated differentials (a methodology performed in most clinical laboratories as part of the CBC) were shown to be unstable at 24 hours. Therefore, if testing is anticipated to be delayed, refrigeration is recommended.

Unrefrigerated EDTA specimens for sedimentation rates should be tested within 4 hours or within 12 hours if the specimens are kept refrigerated (8). Reticulocyte counts drawn into EDTA tubes are considered stable for up to 6 hours at room temperature, 72 hours if kept refrigerated (9).

BOX 6.3	Analytes That Are Unstable at Room Temperature Irrespective of Contact with Cells

- Ammonia
- Acid phosphatase (ACP)
- Coagulation studies (aPTT, PT,* fibrinogen, factor assays, etc.)
- Ethanol*

- Gastrin
- Lactic acid
- Parathyroid hormone (PTH)
- Renin

*After tube has been opened

Because these tests require whole blood, lavender top tubes should not be centrifuged.

Add-On Tests

A working knowledge of analyte stability must be applied by those who process specimens when receiving calls from physicians or their staffs to add tests to previously drawn specimens. *It is not possible to accommodate all requests to add tests to previously collected specimens.* For example, if a lavender top tube was drawn on a hospitalized patient during the morning draw for a CBC and a request to add a reticulocyte count is received later that afternoon, the individual who handles the request should not assume that it can be done. If the tube has been out all day at room temperature, as is the case in most laboratories, a reticulocyte count may not be accurate. In such cases, a fresh specimen must be collected. Failure to apply the knowledge of analyte stability when additional tests are requested for previously drawn specimens puts the patient at risk of being treated or diagnosed according to an incorrect result.

 Tips from the Trenches: *It is not possible to accommodate all requests to add tests to previously collected specimens. (See Table 6.2.)*

Effects of Light

Some analytes deteriorate when exposed to light (Fig. 6.5). The most commonly encountered light-sensitive analyte is bilirubin, which has been shown to undergo up to a 50% reduction in concentration when exposed to light for 1 hour (11). Other light-sensitive analytes include carotene, redblood cell count folate, and vitamin B12. When testing for these constituents, the specimen can be shielded from light during handling, storage, and transport by transferring the serum or plasma into a brown or light restrictive transport tube or by wrapping the specimen in aluminum foil or encasing it in a light-tight transport canister.

It Could Happen to You

A combative patient came to the emergency department (ED) at a large university-based hospital. The nurse drew blood specimens while starting an intravenous (IV) line and sent them to the laboratory. Although the laboratory reported a hemoglobin result of 5.6, the patient demonstrated no clinical signs of anemia or acute blood loss. A repeat CBC was ordered 2 hours later and showed a hemoglobin of 13.6.

Question: How is it possible for a patient to go from a hemoglobin of 5.6 to 13.6 in 2 hours?

Answer: The 5.6 hemoglobin report was the result of a preanalytical error. The ED nurse collected the specimen in a syringe while starting an IV on the patient. After filling the syringe, he set it aside and tended to the IV fluids. At an indeterminate time later, the syringe was evacuated into the tubes and sent to the lab. Significant clotting had likely occurred while the blood sat in the syringe, but not enough to interfere with evacuating a portion of the specimen into the CBC tube. Because a clot had likely formed in the syringe, the specimen evacuated into the tube no longer represented the patient's circulating red blood cell concentration and was not capable of rendering the patient's actual hemoglobin concentration upon testing.

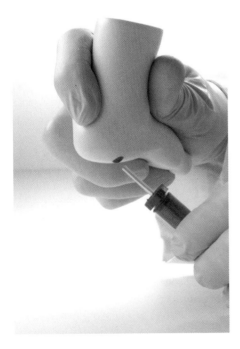

FIGURE 6.5 Protect specimens to be tested for bilirubin from the deteriorating effects of light.

STORAGE AND TRANSPORTATION

On-Site Testing Facilities

When specimens are to be processed and tested within the same physical facility in which they are collected, timely transport is usually not a problem. Those who draw specimens within the facility should adhere to the laboratory's requirements to preserve analyte stability, especially in regard to serum:cell contact and the effects of light on light-sensitive analytes, such as bilirubin. Those who process specimens drawn throughout the facility should be mindful of the deteriorating effects of time, light, and temperature and process all specimens in a timely manner.

Off-Site Testing Facilities

Testing facilities that are remote to the drawing station or patient location present unique challenges to those with blood processing and/or transportation responsibilities. When specimens are drawn in clinics, long-term care facilities, patients' homes, and other settings remote to the testing facility, how the specimen is stored and/or prepared for transportation determines how closely the test results will reflect the patient's condition. To prevent sample deterioration and alteration, proper storage and transportation of the specimen are essential whenever delayed testing is anticipated. Depending upon the test(s) ordered on specimens awaiting transport, some processing steps might be necessary to preserve the analytes to be tested.

 Tips from the Trenches: When specimens are drawn in clinics, long-term care facilities, patients' homes, and other settings remote to the testing facility, how the specimen is stored and/or prepared for transportation determines how closely the test results will reflect the patient's condition.

 Tips from the Trenches: If processing specimens for transportation to testing facilities remote to the drawing site, nonadditive plastic transfer tubes with caps should be available from the testing laboratory for transferring serum.

Adherence to basic specimen handling guidelines will preserve specimen integrity in most specimens. Keeping in mind that there are exceptions, general guidelines can be summarized as follows:

EDTA Tubes

- When collected for CBCs, room temperature storage is acceptable if testing will take place within 24 hours. However, automated differentials may be affected. Refer to the recommendations of the testing facility if prolonged delays in testing are anticipated.

■ When collecting for sedimentation rates, refrigerate specimens if it is anticipated that testing will not take place within 4 hours. Under refrigeration, sedimentation rates are stable for 12 hours.

■ Lavender top tubes collected for reticulocyte counts are stable for 6 hours when kept refrigerated.

■ If testing delays mandate refrigeration during storage prior to transportation, refrigerated temperatures should likewise be maintained during transit.

■ Avoid placing refrigerated specimens in direct contact with ice or other such cooling materials, especially dry ice, as such extremes may cause specimen hemolysis.

Serum Tubes

The concentration of many analytes changes significantly when serum or plasma is exposed to RBCs for prolonged periods of time (Table 6.2) (see "Preventing Glycolysis and Ion Exchange," earlier in this chapter). When it is anticipated that testing blood collected in red stopper tubes or other tubes in which clotting takes place will be delayed beyond 2 hours, allow 20 to 30 minutes for complete clotting to take place (at room temperature), then centrifuge the specimen at the rcf established by the tube manufacturer.

■ Serum must be removed from the RBCs preferably within 1 hour, but no longer than 2 hours after collection, and stored according to the test requirements (3).

■ If the tube does not contain a gel separator, separation can be accomplished by transferring the serum or plasma into a separate transfer tube.

■ Separated serum can be stored at room temperature for up to 8 hours without compromising the stability of most analytes (3). However, because some analytes deteriorate rapidly at room temperature (see Table 6.2), when a delay in transportation and/or testing is anticipated, immediate processing is essential to maintain specimen integrity. Centrifugation should begin immediately after complete clotting has taken place, and the serum should be separated and refrigerated within 2 hours pending transportation to the testing facility.

Heparin Tubes

Whole blood specimens in green top tubes are not to be chilled while waiting for transport to the testing facility unless it is documented that immediate chilling is necessary to preserve the value of the test to be performed (e.g., esoteric tests) (3). These qualifying specimens should be cooled immediately by placing the specimen in a container of crushed ice or ice water after it is collected and labeled. When collecting specimens for potassium (or profiles that include potassium) in conjunction with tests that require specimens to be immediately chilled without centrifugation, a second tube should be collected for the potassium and kept at room temperature. For most other analytes, processing requirements for green top tubes are the same as serum tubes.

Sodium Citrate Tubes

Because many clotting factors deteriorate within hours of collection, it is critical that blue stoppered tubes be processed and tested appropriately. Prothrombin (PT) results can be reliable in an unrefrigerated, uncentrifuged specimen for up to 24 hours after collection. However, aPTTs deteriorate within 4 hours, regardless of temperature or storage conditions. The difference in aPTT results from improper storage and delayed testing is significant and could impact the way the physician medicates the patient. If the medication is based on erroneous results generated from a specimen that was improperly handled and processed, those involved in the specimen handling will have put the patient at risk should the physician adjust the patient's blood thinner based on inaccurate results.

Specimen Processing Reminders

- If specimen testing on serum or plasma is to be delayed beyond 2 hours, the serum or plasma should be separated from the cells by centrifugation and removed from contact with RBCs.
- If the specimen was collected in a gel-separator tube, centrifugation alone will accomplish serum separation, provided centrifugation is adequate and complete clotting has been allowed to occur.
- Tubes with gel separators should not be used on tricyclic antidepressants, progesterone, ionized calcium, and some therapeutic drugs (TDMs). However, affected TDMs depend on the tube's manufacturer. The testing facility should be aware of the limitations of the tubes in use.
- If the tube does not contain a gel separator, the serum/plasma should be removed from the cells within 2 hours of centrifugation, placed into a separate transfer tube, and stored at the appropriate temperature according to the test criteria.
- If the test ordered is an aPTT, the blue top tube should be tested within 4 hours of collection.
- If the patient is on unfractionated heparin therapy, the blue top tube should be centrifuged and the plasma separated from the cells within 1 hour of collection and tested within 4 hours of collection.
- If the test ordered is for a CBC or other hematologic studies, the uncentrifuged lavender top specimen should be refrigerated if testing is to be delayed longer than 4 hours.

Because the storage temperature of the separated serum or plasma is dependent on the analyte being tested, the entire battery of tests ordered must be considered when determining proper storage and transport temperatures and conditions. Whenever the tests ordered require different storage conditions, drawing extra tubes or dividing the serum/plasma into separate fractions may be necessary so that all blood values can be appropriately preserved. The testing facility should provide those who draw specimens that require transportation with a desk reference containing specific information on storage and handling for each test.

A race against time begins the moment blood leaves the body. The ultimate goal is to test the concentration of decaying analytes while they still represent the patient's condition. Phlebotomists and other healthcare professionals who know the affects of time, temperature, and light on test results play a major role in winning that race.

IN THE LAB

Why Do Some Tests Take So Long?

There are many variables in clinical laboratory testing that affect the lab's ability to put out results in a timely manner. Staffing shortages, equipment malfunctions, missing specimens and orders, unverifiable results, communication snafus, and many other avoidable and unavoidable events can bring the testing and reporting process to a screeching halt. However, some delays are legitimate—that is, an inherent element of clinical laboratory testing—and cannot be hastened.

Two of the most frequent legitimate delays are associated with "timed tests" and "send-outs." Timed tests are those that require a fixed amount of time to render results. Not all tests provide instantaneous results. Some incorporate incubation phases, while others require the serum to undergo a time-consuming pretreatment step to eliminate interfering factors. Although robotics and computerized automation continue to shorten the "turnaround time" for lab tests, some functions simply cannot be shortened. For example, blood cultures cannot be finalized as negative until they are allowed to incubate for 5 days. Although preliminary reports are issued, it is unreasonable to expect the first preliminary result until the culture has been allowed to incubate at least 12 hours. Bacteria need at least that much time to multiply to detectable levels. Immediate Gram's stains of blood culture specimens, however, are usually performed within minutes and can serve as a preliminary result.

Sedimentation rates measure how far RBCs will settle in 1 hour when mixed with saline and placed upright in a column. In certain disease states and inflammation, they fall rapidly. Because the results are measured in millimeters per hour, it takes an hour of settling to make the determination. Some systems are in use in clinical laboratories that anticipate the sedimentation rate within 20 minutes. However, since this test is time-dependent, at least a 20-minute delay is inevitable before results can be reported.

All laboratories have to rely to some extent on reference labs to perform those tests for which a low volume of orders makes it impractical to perform in-house. There are well over 1,000 tests that can be performed on blood; no laboratory can do them all. Every testing facility, therefore, has its own list of "send-outs." Depending on the test ordered, the reference lab with which the on-site testing facility contracts to perform infrequently ordered or "esoteric" tests can be across the street, across town, or across the country. Naturally, the farther away the reference lab is, the longer it will take to obtain results. Fortunately, the results of such esoteric tests usually are not needed immediately, yet they provide important information to assist in the diagnosis and long-term management of the patient.

REFERENCES

1. Zhang D Elswick R, Miller W, et al. Effect of serum-clot contact time on clinical chemistry laboratory results. *Clin Chem* 1998;44:1325–1333.
2. Narayanan S. The preanalytic phase: an important component of laboratory medicine. *Am J Clin Pathol* 2000;113:429–452.
3. NCCLS. *Procedures for the handling and processing of blood specimens.* Approved Standard H18-A3.Wayne, PA, 2004.
4. Dasgupta A, Dean, R, Saldana S, et al. Absorption of therapeutic drugs by barrier gels in serum separator blood collection tubes. *Clin Chem* 1993;101:456–461.
5. US Department of Labor and Occupational Safety and Health Administration (OSHA). Occupational exposure to bloodborne pathogens: final rule (29 CFR 1910.1030). *Federal Register* 1991;Dec 6:64004–64182.
6. NCCLS. *Collection, transport, and processing of blood specimens for testing plasma-based coagulation assays.* Approved Standard. H21-A4. Wayne, PA, 2003.
7. Young D. *Effects of preanalytical variables on clinical laboratory tests,* 2nd ed. Washington, DC: AACC Press, 1997.
8. Wintrobe MM. *Wintrobe's Clinical hematology,* 9th ed. Philadelphia: Lea & Febiger, 1993.
9. Koepke J. Update on reticulocyte counting. *Lab Med* 1999;30(5):339–343.
10. Gulati G, Hyland L, Kocher W, et al. Changes in automated complete blood cell count and differential leukocyte count results induced by storage of blood at room temperature. *Arch Pathol Lab Med* 2002;126:336–342.
11. Kiechle F. Q&A response. *Cap Today* 1998;16(4):102–103.

REVIEW QUESTIONS

1. All of the following are specimen-processing errors that can alter patient results except:
   a. misidentifying a patient
   b. improper centrifugation
   c. respinning gel-separator tubes
   d. transporting specimens on ice

2. Most specimens drawn near to the testing lab can be transported at room temperature unless:
   a. the test requires immediate chilling of the specimen
   b. the tube is underfilled
   c. the tube requires centrifugation
   d. the specimen is transported in a pneumatic tube system

3. To preserve analyte stability during transport to remote testing facilities, those who collect and process specimens must take into consideration:
   a. the blood:anticoagulant ratio
   b. the temperature of the transport environment
   c. the analyte's stability over time
   d. b and c

4. To preserve specimen integrity of chemistry analytes, it is of primary importance for:
   a. tubes to be completely filled
   b. serum or plasma to be separated from the cells within 2 hours of collection
   c. specimens to be tested within 4 hours
   d. centrifugation speed to be maintained below 1,500 rpm

5. It is important to assure that blue stoppered (citrate) tubes are transported and tested within 4 hours if:
   a. an activated partial thromboplastin time (aPTT) is to be performed on the specimen
   b. the specimen cannot be immediately centrifuged
   c. the specimen can be immediately centrifuged
   d. a prothrombin (PT) time is to be performed on the specimen

6. As long as serum or plasma remains in contact with red blood cells:
   a. all analytes will remain stable
   b. clotting will occur
   c. significant and irreversible changes take place for all analytes
   d. significant and irreversible changes take place for many analytes

7. According to the Clinical and Laboratory Standards Institute, serum or plasma should be separated from the cells within 2 hours unless:
   a. the specimen can be immediately refrigerated
   b. the specimen contains a clot activator
   c. evidence exists that longer contact times do not contribute to the inaccuracy of the result
   d. a and b

8. For complete blood counts (CBCs), EDTA tubes can be refrigerated:
   a. up to 24 hours without affecting cell counts or morphology
   b. up to 8 hours without affecting cell counts or morphology
   c. up to 4 hours without affecting cell counts or morphology
   d. up to 48 hours without affecting cell counts or morphology
9. For sedimentation rates, EDTA specimens should be:
   a. tested within 2 hours
   b. tested within 4 hours if not refrigerated
   c. tested within 12 hours if kept refrigerated
   d. b and c
10. Reticulocyte counts drawn into EDTA tubes are:
    a. stable for up to 6 hours at room temperature
    b. stable for 72 hours if kept refrigerated
    c. not stable unless centrifuged within 2 hours
    d. a and b
11. Bilirubin can deteriorate up to 50% after:
    a. 2 hours of exposure to light
    b. 1 hour of exposure to light
    c. centrifugation
    d. refrigeration
12. Complete clotting can take up to:
    a. 30 minutes
    b. 2 hours
    c. 30 minutes if refrigerated
    d. 10 minutes
13. Respinning gel tubes that have been stored:
    a. can yield an altered result
    b. should be conducted if more serum is required
    c. will hemolyze cells if the specimen has been refrigerated
    d. should only be conducted on tubes with additives

Phlebotomy Liability 7

INTRODUCTION

Phlebotomy is an invasive procedure with risks to the patient when performed improperly. Among those risks are permanent and disabling nerve injuries, arterial laceration, uncontrolled hemorrhaging, injuries from loss of consciousness, and complications from improperly identified patients and specimens. In this chapter, insights will be offered into how those who collect blood specimens and their employers can be liable for injuries inflicted during the procedure. Case studies of patients injured during blood collection procedures will be used to illustrate steps of the process that, when neglected or performed haphazardly, can not only result in permanent injury or death to the patient, but subject the individual who performed the procedure and his/her employer to a firestorm of litigation. Strategies that prevent liability for phlebotomy-related injuries will be discussed with the objective of limiting healthcare personnel's vulnerability to inflicting injuries that lead to litigation.

Upon completion of this chapter, the reader should be able to:

- Identify the most common injuries poor phlebotomy technique inflicts upon patients
- Associate errors in technique, judgment, and supervision with phlebotomy-related injuries
- Describe the anatomy of the antecubital area in regard to nerves, veins, and the brachial artery
- Discuss the risks involved when attempting to access the basilic vein

PHLEBOTOMY LIABILITY

Every year thousands of patients are injured during venipuncture procedures. Some injuries resolve, some are permanent. The presence of nerves, tendons, and arteries in the antecubital area present a risk that cannot be eliminated even by the most skilled phlebotomist. Many occur even when the procedure is performed correctly. However, most injuries occur because the healthcare personnel performing the procedure failed to fully appreciate the risk and performed the procedure against the established standards. In a legal context, performing a procedure against the prevailing and acceptable standards is referred to as performing beneath the "standard of care." Should it be found that performing beneath the standard of care resulted in an injury to the patient, the cost to the employer can be in the tens or hundreds of thousands of dollars in legal fees, compensation, and punitive damages. The cost to the patient is incalculable.

The only way to avoid legal liability is to know the standard of care for blood specimen collection and operate within it at all times.

Standard of Care

The standard of care is loosely defined as *what a reasonable and prudent phlebotomist would have done under similar circumstances.* The premise is that a reasonable and prudent phlebotomist is adequately trained according to the prevailing standard and performs the procedure according to that standard at all times. If evidence emerges that critical aspects and precautions might have been abandoned, the attorneys engage in a spirited debate to prove or disprove negligence. Depending upon the success of either side to advance their argument, the case may or may not be settled out of court.

Typically, once an injury occurs, patients allow time for it to resolve. Depending on the nature and extent of the injury, medical treatment may be sought immediately. As long-term consequences of the injury become evident, patients may be moved to seek legal representation to collect damages for any pain, suffering, and/or disability the injury may have caused and to recover lost wages and any medical expenses incurred. Once an attorney is retained, a standard sequence of events is set into motion to ultimately answer one question: "Was the procedure performed within the standard of care?"

To make this determination, the patient's attorney will research how venipunctures ought to be performed when they are performed properly given the unique circumstances of the case. Not only is the standard of care for the procedure researched, but the standard of care for the training and evaluation of individuals who perform blood collection procedures will be explored. Both of these processes are accomplished by reviewing textbooks, articles, and published standards and by consulting with authorities in the field (Fig. 7.1).

While the patient's attorney researches the standard of care for the procedure, he/she concurrently attempts to reconstruct how the procedure was actually performed. This is accomplished through a series of interviews with those involved. These interviews can be informal—as in private conversations between attorney and client—or in the form of a "deposition." A deposition is a formal question/answer session between the attorney and witness (e.g., patient, phlebotomist, supervisor, etc.) in the presence of a court reporter. Anyone involved in the case can be deposed. Through a series of probing questions conducted under oath during the deposition, the attorney seeks to establish a first-

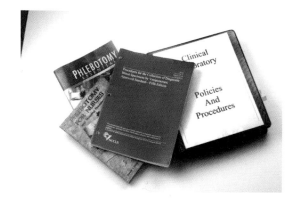

FIGURE 7.1 The only way to avoid legal liability is to know what the standard of care is for blood specimen collection and operate within it at all times.

hand account of the individual's involvement in the incident that led to the injury. All information rendered becomes admissible in court as evidence.

While researching the standard of care, the patient's attorney simultaneously attempts to establish hard evidence that an injury has occurred, i.e., evidence that an injury has taken place beyond the patient's own claim of pain or complications resulting from the puncture. Unlike whiplash injuries from auto accidents, most phlebotomy-related injuries can be proved or disproved by medical examinations and tests. If the injury cannot be documented, the case can still proceed. However, from an attorney's perspective, a case in which there is documented evidence that an injury has occurred is more inviting and easier to pursue.

Should the patient's attorney's research reveal the case has merit, a complaint or suit usually is filed against the employer of the individual who performed the procedure. Rarely is the employee named in the lawsuit because of (1) the limited potential to collect the damages sought and (2) the employer's responsibility to the patient that the staff is adequately trained and supervised to prevent injuries. When notified of the legal action being taken, the employer's attorney conducts the same research to determine the standard of care pertinent to the case and the circumstances surrounding the procedure.

If evidence indicates some procedural deviations may have put the patient at risk, the answer to a second question is sought concurrently: "Did the person responsible for the training and evaluation of the individual performing the venipuncture put the patient at risk by improperly managing the employee?" Attorneys on both sides go to great lengths searching for evidence that will answer these pivotal questions in their favor. Employment records containing information on the hiring, training, evaluation, and disciplining of the employee can be subpoenaed as evidence to prove or disprove that inadequate employee management contributed to the injury. The facility's procedure manual also can be scrutinized to see if it is consistent with the prevailing standard or if the employee deviated from the facility's procedure. Failure to follow an established procedure reflecting the prevailing standard often results in charges that the facility failed to adequately evaluate and/or discipline the employee for violating facility policy.

As the process unfolds, each side acts as if it will eventually have to present a convincing case to a jury. If the patient's attorney can find convincing evidence that the individual or facility violated the standard of care and by so doing contributed to an injury, hopes are raised that a jury will find the facility liable. Likewise, if the facility's (defense) attorney can convincingly prove that no violations in the standard of care exist, it raises hopes that the jury will exonerate the facility, releasing it from liability. If the case substantially weakens for either side during the process, the case is dropped or an out-of-court settlement is reached. In most cases, the evidence that emerges provides obstacles for one side or another and the case is settled without going to trial.

However, should the case proceed, any employee—however remotely linked to the procedure or the individual who performed it—may be called as a witness. It is critical, therefore, for all healthcare personnel to know what the standard states about the procedure as it relates to the case being tried and not to testify against it. Those who are aware of the standard of care for phlebotomy can avoid the embarrassment and anxiety on the witness stand that can ensue when the attorney knows more about the procedure than the witness does.

 Tips from the Trenches: *If called to testify in a phlebotomy-related injury case, healthcare personnel should know what the standard states about the procedure and not testify against it.*

For those who perform phlebotomy, the only way to avoid the anxiety of depositions and court testimony is to learn to draw a blood specimen according to the standards set forth by the Clinical and Laboratory Standards Institute, the literature, and the facility's procedure manual and to apply this knowledge every time. A regular review of these documents is important to maintain compliance.

Injuries that Bring Lawsuits

It's important to realize that just because a patient is injured during a blood collection procedure, it doesn't mean the individual who performed the procedure did something wrong to contribute to the injury. Phlebotomy is an invasive procedure with risks. Those who are properly trained and supervised and who perform within the standard of care reduce this risk to its lowest possible degree. But the risk can never be completely eliminated. Unfortunately, most injuries inflicted by healthcare personnel during blood collection procedures occur because of one or more deviations from the standard of care.

Injuries that patients typically suffer that prompt legal action include:

- Nerve injury
- Hemorrhage from arterial nick
- Hemorrhage from inadequate pressure to the vein
- Complications from drawing from the same side as a mastectomy
- Injuries sustained from syncope during a phlebotomy procedure

It Could Happen to You

During a trial involving a phlebotomy-related nerve injury, the phlebotomist's supervisor testified that a 40-degree angle of insertion was an acceptable angle. The patient's attorney cited publication after publication stating a 15- to 30-degree angle of insertion was the norm, yet the supervisor continued to testify that an angle beyond that stated in the published literature was acceptable at their facility. Finally, the attorney read from the laboratory's own procedure manual, which reflected the literature.

Question: What could the supervisor have done to prevent being humiliated on the witness stand?

Answer: Clearly the supervisor was unaware of what the standards reflected in regard to the angle of insertion. Had she properly researched the standards, she would have likely realized that the phlebotomist performed beneath the standard of care without justification and should have advised the facility's attorney to settle out of court. Instead, the patient's attorney built a convincing case that the facility considered itself immune from the standard of care, even from their own procedures, by supporting an angle of insertion greater than 30 degrees.

Nerve Injuries

Most healthcare personnel with blood collection responsibilities are aware of the location of the three veins in the antecubital area suitable for venipuncture. Most also know the location of the brachial artery. Unfortunately, few are aware of where nerves pass through the area and how to avoid them. Nerves are neither visible nor palpable. Therefore, those who are not aware of their location in the antecubital area are not aware of how to reduce the risk of nerve injury to its lowest possible degree. (See illustration of the anatomy of the antecubital area in Chapter 3.)

Documentation of a nerve injury alone is not sufficient proof a deviation from the standard of care has occurred. Injury alone does not automatically impart liability. In order for liability to be ascribed, it must be shown that the procedure was performed beneath the standard of care. Even the most skilled phlebotomist can injure a nerve while operating within the standard of care. This is largely due to the fact that the nerves pass precariously close to the basilic vein, an acceptable vein for specimen collection. Because the needle disappears beneath the surface of the skin, phlebotomists are left with their mind's eye to guide the needle tip into the vein. A thorough knowledge of the anatomy of the antecubital area sharpens the visualization of needle placement, but individual variations in anatomy are inevitable. Careful site selection and limited needle relocation helps prevent injury.

 Tips from the Trenches: *Nerve injuries are one of the most common injuries that occur when the procedure is not performed according to the standards.*

Arterial Nicks

The proximity of the brachial artery to the basilic vein also makes punctures to this vein risky. As discussed under "Technical Errors," later in this chapter, attempts to access the basilic vein may not be justified if it can be shown that a medial or cephalic vein was available at the time. The most common errors in technique that involve the brachial artery are an excessive angle of insertion and excessive probing. Nicks to the brachial artery are not always evident and if undetected can lead to hemorrhaging long after the puncture has been completed. If blood accumulates in the affected arm, the pressure can result in a compression nerve injury or, in extreme circumstances, require emergency surgery to repair a laceration and/or remove muscle fascia.

Before inserting the needle in an attempt to access the basilic vein, collectors must ascertain the location of the brachial artery and avoid needle placement that may puncture or nick the structure. Once located, the needle can be inserted only if there is confidence that the artery can be avoided. Should the basilic vein not be accessed upon needle insertion, side-to-side needle relocation should not be attempted (1). Do not attempt to access the basilic vein if the brachial artery is too close to be sure it can be avoided.

When inserting the needle into this area, collectors must observe for the signs of an arterial nick for the duration of the venipuncture and after the needle is removed (i.e., bright red blood and/or rapid hematoma formation) (Fig. 7.2). Should any of these signs be observed, discontinue the draw immediately and apply at least 5 minutes of pressure (1). Failure to detect these signs and react appropriately puts the patient and facility at risk.

 Tips from the Trenches: Should the basilic vein not be accessed upon needle insertion, side-to-side needle relocation should not be attempted.

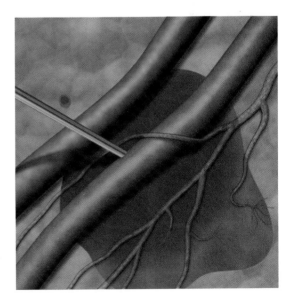

FIGURE 7.2 When inserting the needle into this area, collectors must observe for the signs of an arterial nick. (From Center for Phlebotomy Education with Permission.)

It Could Happen to You

A nurse at a blood donor station attempted to obtain a unit of blood from a basilic vein that was palpable, but not visible. Initially unsuccessful at accessing the vein, she attempted to manipulate the 16-gauge needle to find the vein and was unsuccessful. The donor was bandaged and sent home. Later in the day he went to the emergency room because his arm had swelled and become intolerably painful. The emergency room physician diagnosed a compression injury to the nerves secondary to an arterial nick that hemorrhaged into his arm. The lingering nerve injury resulted in a lawsuit against the facility.

Question: How could the nurse have prevented the injury?

Answer: Clearly, one or more of the nurse's probing motions punctured the brachial artery. Had she recognized the potential for needle manipulation in the area of the basilic vein to pierce the brachial artery or nerves, she would not have relocated the needle. A potential second error is that she may not have taken adequate time to observe the puncture site for hematoma formation before bandaging. The reasonable and prudent healthcare professional does not relocate the needle in the area of the basilic vein and takes time to observe for subcutaneous bleeding before bandaging.

Venous Hemorrhage

Many patients have suffered permanent injuries because the individual performing the venipuncture failed to apply adequate pressure after the puncture to ensure that bleeding had stopped.

 According to the Standards . . . check that bleeding has ceased, observe for hematoma, and apply an adhesive or gauze bandage over the venipuncture site.

It Could Happen to You

A patient entered an outpatient drawing station of a laboratory. The phlebotomist failed to initially access the vein, probed several times in the area of the brachial artery, and eventually obtained the specimen. Upon needle removal, the patient applied pressure. The phlebotomist eventually bandaged the site without lifting the gauze to check for bleeding. Within moments the patient's upper arm became grotesquely swollen and she was rushed to a physician's office where an arterial hemorrhage was detected. The hemorrhage exerted pressure on the nerves in the area and the patient developed a permanently disabling injury to the arm.

Question: How could this hemorrhage have been avoided?

Answer: This injury occurred because the phlebotomist probed in the area of the brachial artery and failed to lift the gauze to observe for superficial bleeding and hematoma formation before bandaging. Had she checked, the rapidly forming hematoma would have been immediately detected and additional pressure applied.

Because it is not always evident which patients have compromised clotting abilities, all patients should be treated as susceptible to prolonged bleeding. It is not sufficient to simply observe for superficial bleeding; collectors should also observe for bleeding that can occur subcutaneously (1). Even though the skin may have closed, the vein may continue to hemorrhage into the tissue. Before bandaging, remove the gauze and watch the puncture site for a few moments to look for a raising or mounding of the tissue indicating the vein has not yet sealed. Apply additional pressure if necessary.

Drawing from Mastectomy Patients

Performing a venipuncture or capillary puncture on the same side as a prior mastectomy without physician's permission goes against Clinical and Laboratory Standards Institute standards (see "Site Selection," Chapter 2, and "Difficult Draws," Chapter 4) (1). The standards issue no exceptions on how long ago the mastectomy was performed or for draws on patients who have had bilateral mastectomies. If a draw from the same side as a mastectomy is the only option, the physician should be notified and given the chance to reduce the tests so that a lesser quantity of blood can be obtained by a capillary puncture on the unaffected side. If there are no other options, the physician's permission must be obtained before venipunctures or capillary punctures to the affected side are attempted. Written permission should be obtained to appoint the proper liability should the patient subsequently seek damages for pain and suffering that can result. Because this restriction is so well documented in the standards and literature, attorneys who seek damages to compensate the patient for pain or suffering usually have an easy case.

 According to the Standards . . . a physician must be consulted before drawing blood by venipuncture or capillary puncture from the same side as a prior mastectomy.

Injuries from Loss of Consciousness

One of the known risks of phlebotomy is the potential for the patient to lose consciousness. A reasonable and prudent phlebotomist knows this, anticipates every patient will pass out, and is prepared to react to prevent injury (Fig. 7.3). Observing for the signs of an imminent loss of consciousness—pallor, perspiration, lightheadedness, hyperventilation, anxiety, dizziness, nausea, etc.—throughout the duration of the procedure and until the patient is released from your care is paramount to preventing, or at least limiting, injuries that can occur. See Chapter 3 on managing patients with vertigo or syncope.

 According to the Standards . . . the use of ammonia inhalants is not recommended.

When reacting to a patient who is feeling faint or who has passed out, avoid the use of ammonia inhalants as some patients may have respiratory disorders such as asthma or emphysema.

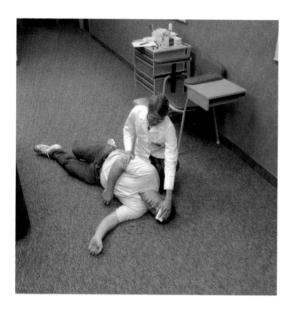

FIGURE 7.3 A reasonable and prudent healthcare worker anticipates every patient will pass out and is prepared to react to prevent injury.

Death

When patients are misidentified or treated according to results that are rendered inaccurate by specimen collection errors, the employer of the individual who performed the specimen collection procedure may be liable for negative patient outcomes, including death. Failure to follow the standard protocol for

It Could Happen to You

A city worker was sent to the local laboratory for random blood and urine drug screens. When he notified the phlebotomist that he has a tendency to pass out when he gets his blood drawn, the phlebotomist suggested he lie down on the bed for the draw. He refused. After several attempts to convince him, the phlebotomist agreed to draw the patient in the drawing chair. She then sent him to the restroom to collect the urine specimen, having obtained verbal and visual assurances that he was not about to pass out. Upon closing the door, he passed out and fractured his skull on the sink.

Question: What could the phlebotomist have done to prevent this injury?

Answer: It could be argued that the patient should have been sent to the restroom before the venipuncture, but it is likely that the syncopal episode still would have occurred, leading to other injuries. It also could be argued that the phlebotomist should have refused to draw the patient in anything other than a recumbent position given her knowledge of his history of passing out during blood draws. Granted, the patient does have some responsibilities to himself and should have complied with the phlebotomist's wishes, but in today's litigious society, rigidly adhering to facility policy would have likely limited the facility's liability.

It Could Happen to You

A medical assistant was sent by her employer to draw blood from a woman in her home who had applied for a life insurance policy. The patient was seated in an armless kitchen chair and the venipuncture was successfully completed. When the medical assistant turned his back to label the tubes and process the application, the applicant passed out, fell to the floor, and fractured a vertebra. She is now paralyzed.

Question: What could the medical assistant have done differently to prevent this injury?

Answer: The medical assistant committed two blatant errors that contributed to this tragic and unnecessary injury. By seating the patient in an armless chair, there was nothing to keep the patient from falling to the floor. The second error was to turn his back on the patient after the draw. The reasonable and prudent healthcare professional recognizes the risk of all patients to pass out and is prepared to protect patients from falls and injuries that can occur.

patient identification and drawing blood above an active intravenous (IV) line are just two types of specimen collection errors that have resulted in patient death.

 Tips from the Trenches: Those who refuse to violate the established protocol are the patient's last line of defense against medical errors that lead to complications and death.

Healthcare personnel with blood specimen collection responsibilities must be aware of the potential for tragic consequences resulting from deviations from the standard procedure. All collection personnel, especially in acute care settings, are inevitably thrust into situations that tempt them to label speci-

It Could Happen to You

Upon admission to the hospital, a patient changed beds with her roommate. The technician who drew her blood for a preop crossmatch failed to perform the proper patient identification procedure and drew blood on her roommate instead. The patient went to surgery, received incompatible blood, and died.

Question: How could this tragic death have been avoided?

Answer: Assuming the patient in the bed was the same patient the test requisition said was in the bed was the dangerous assumption that precipitated this tragedy. Had the patient's identification bracelet been checked and confirmed against the patient's verbal response to the question "what is your name?" the discrepancy probably would have been identified and corrected.

mens drawn by other healthcare personnel, label specimens after leaving the patient's side, and make assumptions on patient identification. Those with the discipline to refuse to violate the established protocol establish themselves as the patient's last line of defense against medical errors that lead to complications and death.

Technical Errors

Blood collection personnel who don't appreciate the risk of the procedure can injure patients in many ways. Some of the most common errors committed include:

- Failure to properly identify the patient. Because this error has the greatest potential to lead to patient death, following the proper protocol for patient identification for every patient without fail is paramount to protecting patients and reducing liability. The Clinical and Laboratory Standards Institute is very clear on the proper means of patient identification (see Chapter 3). Yet many situations arise in healthcare settings that challenge specimen collection personnel to make assumptions and cut corners for convenience and expediency. It takes discipline and a dedication to the patient and facility protocol to properly protect patients from life-threatening errors.
- Poor vein selection. To reduce the risk of injury, collectors must perform a thorough survey of the antecubital areas of both arms in search of an acceptable medial or cephalic vein prior to performing a puncture to the basilic vein (Fig. 7.4). It is well established in the standards and the literature that the basilic vein lies in close proximity to the nerves that pass through the antecubital area, establishing it as the vein with the greatest risk of injury to the patient (1–5). Not only can the nerves pass alongside of the basilic vein, but they can cross over it as well (2). If it can be shown the collector failed to perform a thorough survey of all available veins or that the collector had the choice of puncturing the medial vein, but chose the basilic vein without justification and subsequently injured the patient, it can be effectively argued that the collector's judgment did not reduce the risk of injury to its lowest possible degree. That is not to say that all punctures must be conducted on the medial or cephalic veins, but it is critical that the collector rule out the safer veins before selecting the basilic vein.
- Poor site selection. Not all veins are fair game. The recognized sites for venipuncture include the antecubital area, the dorsal side of the hand, and the lateral side of the wrist. Feet and ankle veins are permitted only with a physician's permission. Draws outside of these areas are unorthodox and may have to be justified should the procedure lead to a patient injury. When performing an invasive procedure such as venipuncture, a thorough knowledge of the anatomy of the area to be punctured is necessary to reduce the risk of injury to its lowest possible degree.

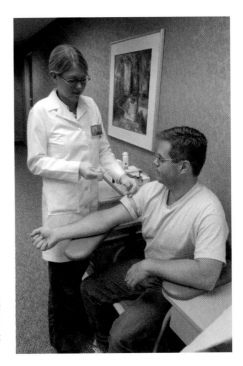

FIGURE 7.4 Collectors must perform a thorough survey of the antecubital areas of both arms for the presence of a medial vein to reduce the risk of injury to its lowest possible degree.

- Excessive angle of insertion. One of the most common errors collectors make that lead to nerve injury is entering the vein at an excessive angle of insertion. When the needle enters the vein obtusely, it is much more likely to pass through the other side of the vein than if entered at a low angle. A long "breaking distance" allows the collector a significant margin of error before emerging through the other side of the vein and potentially injuring underlying structures. Unless extenuating circumstances justify an excessive angle, insert the needle at an angle of 30 degrees or less (1,3–6).

It Could Happen to You

A gentleman entered a blood donor facility to donate a unit of blood. Having selected the basilic vein and failing to access it on needle insertion, the nurse began probing with a 16-gauge needle, eventually piercing the median nerve and causing permanent damage. The donor filed a lawsuit against the blood donation facility for the injury.

Question: How could the nurse have avoided injuring the donor?

Answer: Probing to relocate a missed vein should never be attempted, especially in the area where the nerves and brachial artery pass. Upon needle insertion and failure to access the vein, the nurse should have removed the needle and attempted to access another vein.

- Excessive probing. Often, the vein is not accessed on needle insertion. The Clinical and Laboratory Standards Institute is very specific on the limits of needle relocation if the vein is not initially accessed (1). A reasonable and prudent phlebotomist attempting to access the basilic vein understands that the nerves and brachial artery lie in close proximity and that any side-to-side needle relocation risks complications that can lead to disabling injuries. Under certain circumstances, a vein's orientation to the needle can be easily corrected by a calculated relocation providing the collector exercises sound professional judgment based on an understanding of the risks and the standards. Such calculated needle relocations should only be attempted while accessing a median or cephalic vein and only if the collector feels confident that it can be conducted safely and successfully. That confidence, however, cannot exist when accessing the basilic vein because of the close proximity of other structures that could be injured. Blindly probing in any area should never be conducted.
- Failure to anticipate syncope. Healthcare personnel with specimen collection responsibilities should not underestimate the potential for all patients to lose consciousness during or immediately following the procedure. Collectors who fail to anticipate syncope may not be in a position to protect the fainting patient from falling and sustaining serious injury. Because it has been estimated that up to 20% of the population has a fear of needles (see Chapter 4), a lack of preparedness can translate to liability should the injuries prompt legal action. To protect patients from injuries that can result from a loss of consciousness, healthcare personnel should take the following precautions when drawing blood from any patient:
    - Outpatients should be drawn from a chair designed for phlebotomy with features that will support the patient on all four sides should he/she lose consciousness. This includes a pivoting arm that locks in front of the patient to provide support for the arm and to prevent forward falls (1).
    - Inpatients, emergency department patients, and patients in clinics and physicians' offices should be reclined on a bed, gurney, or examination table or seated in a chair with side supports
    - Patients drawn in their homes by visiting nurses, medical assistants, or other allied healthcare personnel including those who draw specimens for insurance purposes should recline the patient in a comfortable position on a bed or sofa or position the patient in a chair with side supports that provide confidence the patient will not fall to the floor if there is a loss of consciousness.
    - Under no circumstances should blood be drawn from a patient sitting upright on an armless chair, bed, cot, gurney, examination table, or any structure without back and side support that can prevent the patient from falling off.
    - Never allow patients to leave your sight until they are released. Directing your attention away from them to label tubes, complete paperwork, deliver specimens, etc. is neglecting the risk of syncope. A

reasonable and prudent phlebotomist recognizes the risk and remains vigilant throughout the entire procedure until the patient is released from his/her care.

- Ask patients if they have ever had a problem with getting their blood drawn. If they indicate they have become lightheaded or have passed out, recline the patient on a bed, cot, or gurney for the procedure.
- Constantly observe the patient throughout the procedure for the signs of vertigo or syncope and be prepared to terminate the procedure before completion. Never attempt to complete the draw during a syncopal episode as seizures may ensue risking injury to both patient and collector.

See Chapter 3 for how to react to a patient who loses consciousness.

- Failure to provide adequate pressure to the puncture site. Just as we must always anticipate that patients may pass out, we must always expect patients to continue bleeding from the puncture after pressure is released. We don't always know when patients are taking a blood thinner or an aspirin every day for their heart. For them, vein and skin closure may be prolonged. The reasonable and prudent phlebotomist makes sure adequate pressure is applied by applying it him-/herself or by allowing the willing patient to assist. If the patient is allowed to apply pressure, the collector is vigilant throughout the postvenipuncture activities, making sure pressure is adequate and not prematurely released. Therefore, while being alert for the signs of vertigo and syncope, observe those patients who are applying pressure to their puncture site to ensure that the pressure is constant and adequate. It is ultimately the phlebotomist's responsibility to ensure that adequate pressure is applied to prevent complications from hematoma formation. Allowing the patient to bend the arm at the elbow is not considered an adequate substitute for pressure.

It Could Happen to You

At a drug rehabilitation facility, nursing assistants escorted a patient to the facility's laboratory for blood work. The patient notified the attendants and the phlebotomist that he usually passes out when he gets his blood drawn. The assistants then left the area. After a successful venipuncture, the phlebotomist visually and verbally checked the patient, felt assured he wasn't going to pass out, then released him to return to his room. As soon as he left the laboratory area, he passed out, fell to the floor, and broke his jaw and his arm. The lawsuit that was filed sought damages for the injuries.

Question: How could this injury have been prevented?

Answer: Positioning the patient on a cot or bed for the draw may have prevented the loss of consciousness, but the most blatant error here was that the patient was allowed to return to his room without being escorted by the nursing assistants who knew he had a history of passing out after a blood test.

- Failure to observe for bleeding and hematoma. As detailed in Chapter 3, the collector must be assured that the punctures to the skin and the vein have sealed before bandaging and releasing the patient. This requires the removal of pressure and a visual observation of a duration that allows the detection of hematoma formation, which indicates the vein has not sealed (1). Five to 10 seconds is usually adequate to conclude the puncture to the skin and vein has sealed (Fig. 7.5). Failure to provide or monitor pressure to the puncture site and to observe for hematoma formation before bandaging can bring liability upon the facility should bleeding occur after the patient is released.
- Failure to label specimens at the patient's side. Any delay in labeling the specimens after they are drawn subjects the patient to the risk of being treated according to the results obtained from another patient's blood. The outcome can be tragic. All who draw blood specimens must discipline themselves to make no exceptions to labeling specimens at the patient's side. Should specimens be removed from the patient's room or immediate proximity, events can unfold that lead to labeling errors. All facilities should adopt a zero tolerance policy for not labeling specimens at the patient's side.
- Accepting unlabeled specimens. When specimens are drawn and then transported from the patient's side unlabeled and handed to another employee or department, they should be discarded and recollected. The risk of misidentifying the specimen is too great when specimen labeling responsibilities are handed off to anyone other than the person who

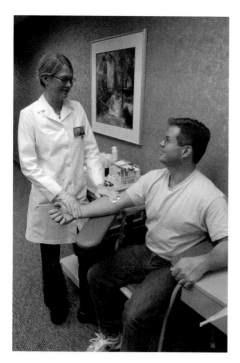

FIGURE 7.5 Before bandaging, apply adequate pressure to the puncture site and observe for hematoma prior to bandaging.

It Could Happen to You

An outpatient came to a small county hospital for his monthly coagulation studies. The phlebotomist drew the blood successfully from his antecubital area, checked the site for visible bleeding, then bandaged and released the patient. However, the patient continued to bleed subcutaneously, resulting in gradual hemorrhaging into the entire extremity, nearly necessitating the amputation of his arm.

Question: How could the phlebotomist have prevented such extensive hemorrhaging?

Answer: Those who perform venipunctures must anticipate prolonged bleeding in all patients and watch for the formation of a hematoma prior to bandaging. Observing for visible bleeding is not enough to assure that the puncture to the vein has sealed. A 5- to 10-second visual observation usually is sufficient to detect a subcutaneous bleed. When recognized, additional pressure is necessary before bandaging and releasing the patient.

drew the specimen. Anyone who accepts an unlabeled specimen and applies the label is assuming the patient was properly identified by the collector. Such assumptions in healthcare can be tragic.

Often, healthcare personnel thrust into situations in which they are asked to label specimens they have not drawn are the patient's last line of defense against medical mistakes that could kill them. Those who uphold policies such as not accepting unlabeled specimens are well-placed allies of patients and of the healthcare facility to which they have entrusted their care.

Administrative Errors

Phlebotomy supervisors, nurse managers, laboratory directors, and human resource managers all have a role to play in protecting patients from phlebotomy-related errors and litigation. If it can be shown that the facility engaged in inadequate hiring, training, and/or evaluation practices regarding the employee involved in a phlebotomy-related injury, it can be argued that the facility failed to protect the patient from unskilled employees.

Training and Evaluation

Those involved in the hiring, training, and evaluation of specimen collection personnel in all departments can best protect the employer from such liability by making sure the policies instituted for all employees with blood collection responsibilities and the manner in which they were implemented can stand up to scrutiny by a jury (see Chapter 1). A training program for those new to specimen collection should be comprehensive and include didactic and practical components. Although California is the only state with minimum training requirements, all employers should establish a training protocol that adequately protects their patients from the unskilled. (See Appendix V, "Minimum Content for Phlebotomy Training Program.")

Regardless of prior experience or training, new employees should be subjected to a period of observation of sufficient duration to thoroughly assess their skills and correct deficiencies in technique (Fig. 7.6). Once cleared for performing without supervision, all employees with specimen collection responsibilities should be evaluated within 3 to 6 months and annually thereafter to assure that their technique continues to reflect the standards and facility policy. Observing a routine venipuncture and skin puncture is recommended (see Appendix V). In addition, an oral or written assessment of the employees' knowledge can reveal lapses in their understanding and comprehension of phlebotomy that cannot be revealed through observation alone. Administrators and supervisors of in-house phlebotomy staff should devise a short quiz that measures cognitive skills that are critical to patient safety and specimen integrity.

However, merely establishing and implementing sound policies directing the hiring, training, and evaluation of specimen collection personnel is not enough. Without proper documentation that the policies were followed (i.e., training was complete, evaluations were thorough and regular, employees committing infractions were disciplined, continuing education was documented, etc.), it may be argued that the drafting of policies was simply an academic exercise for the benefit of inspectors and that the administrator's failure to implement policies and enforce procedures put the patient population at risk. In legal proceedings, policies and procedures may as well not exist if it can't be shown that they were routinely followed. All those managing specimen collection personnel should make sure that the policies in effect in their facilities regarding hiring, training, and evaluation are adequate and implemented.

 Tips from the Trenches: *Those involved in the hiring, training, and evaluation of specimen collection personnel can protect the employer from liability by making sure that policies and their implementation can stand up to scrutiny.*

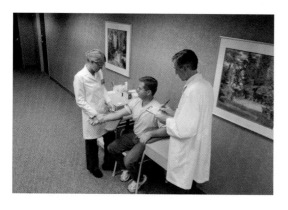

FIGURE 7.6 Observing each employee's routine venipuncture and skin puncture technique annually helps assure that the staff's skills continue to reflect the standards and facility policy.

Giving a Deposition

(From *Ernst D, Ernst C. Phlebotomy for nurses and nursing personnel. Ramsey IN: Healthstar Press, 2001.*)

Depositions are used to set forth admissible evidence that either supports or refutes accusations of liability. Healthcare professionals who are called on to give an account of their involvement in an incident that allegedly resulted in an injury should be prepared to respond to probing questions about any and all aspects of their credentials, job responsibilities, involvement in the case, and recollection of the incident. It is best to begin preparing for a deposition as soon as it becomes evident that the patient is pursuing legal proceedings. Accusations can take place long after the incident that caused them. Regardless of the time that has passed since the incident took place, healthcare professionals involved should attempt to reconstruct the event through memory and such documents.

A deposition can be held in any location convenient to all participating parties (a conference room at the facility, an attorney's office, etc.) and typically involves the questioning of a key witness in the presence of one or both attorneys and a court reporter. It is possible that the patient and/or the facility's risk manager also will be present as an observer.

The deposition will begin with the witness taking the oath to tell the truth, followed by introductory remarks by the questioning attorney to define and clarify the process for the witness and establish basic ground rules for answering questions. For the record, the witness will be asked to identify him-/herself and provide a brief personal history. The questioning attorney will then attempt to reconstruct the witness's involvement in the case to capture on record any deviations from the standard of care or release the witness from liability, depending on the objective of the questioning attorney. If the questioning is being conducted by the patient's attorney, the facility's attorney should be present to assure that proper procedures are followed and that the questioning attorney doesn't use unethical tactics; intimidating lines of questioning; or otherwise offend, confuse, or abuse the witness.

During the course of the deposition, it is critical that the witness maintains composure and answers the questions truthfully and to the best of his/her knowledge. The answers issued during the deposition become admissible in court. Therefore, it is best not to speculate on the details of the case. Because the deposition can take place months or years after the incident, many facts will simply be forgotten or become vague recollections at best. Avoid temptations to reconstruct the incident based on presumptions, assumptions, and speculation. Questions that attempt to establish a fact about an aspect of the incident with which witnesses are uncertain should be answered with "I don't know," "I don't remember," "I can't respond to that with certainty," etc.

Depositions can be gut-wrenching, especially if the facts that come out establish guilt or reveal deviations from the standard of care. The role of the witness in the deposition is not to exonerate oneself or one's employer, but to uncover the truth. If there have been transgressions from the standard procedure or in training/evaluation practices, they should come to light. Only through pursuit of the truth can justice be served and a facility benefit from the exposure of lapses in their policies and procedures, thereby preventing future injuries.

If there is any indication that the patient suffered an injury during the puncture, healthcare professionals who take the time at the moment to record every aspect of the venipuncture for future reference will save themselves immeasurable anxiety when attempting to reconstruct the events.

A Tragedy of Errors

(From *Ernst D.* Avoiding Phlebotomy-Related Lawsuits. 2004 © American Society for Clinical Pathology. Tech Sample is an annual continuing education program for technologists, technicians, and phlebotomists. Reproduced with permission.)

A 51-year-old male comes to the laboratory outpatient desk to have his blood drawn for routine lab work. The phlebotomist looks at his papers and asks, "Are you Howard Miller?" The patient nods affirmatively. The phlebotomist was recently hired directly from a vocational training program where she completed a 6-month phlebotomy course. Even though the facility's policy states that all new phlebotomists must undergo 40 hours of supervision, the phlebotomist's technique so impressed her supervisor that after 3 hours of observation, she was cleared to draw specimens unsupervised.

The phlebotomist seated the patient in the outpatient drawing chair and tightened the tourniquet. She located the basilic vein by palpation on the inside aspect of the antecubital area, loosened the tourniquet, assembled her equipment, and put on gloves. She retightened the tourniquet, relocated the vein, cleansed the site, and performed the puncture using a tube holder/needle assembly. However, when no blood was obtained upon applying the first tube, the phlebotomist removed the tube, relocated the needle, and reapplied the tube without success. She made several more attempts to relocate the needle without accessing the vein. Suddenly the patient felt shooting pain in the limb from the needle insertion point to his fingertips; his arm jumped violently and he shouted in excruciating pain. The phlebotomist apologized, but continued to probe for the vein to the objection of the patient. The pain worsened, but the phlebotomist continued, eventually obtaining a blood specimen and completing the procedure.

Upon needle removal, she instructed the patient to apply pressure while she labeled the specimens. She bandaged the site without checking for bleeding and apologized to the patient who looked pale and was perspiring. Embarrassed by the pain her technique brought to the patient, she hastened out of the room with the specimens. The patient attempted to get out of the chair to leave the outpatient drawing area and collapsed on the floor. His arm began to rapidly swell at the puncture site. His fall was observed by other phlebotomists, and the patient was revived and sent to the emergency room for treatment and evaluation.

The patient's specimen was taken to the lab and tested for coagulation studies. The results showed that he was overmedicated with heparin, prompting the technician to report the result to the physician. The physician immediately called the patient, Howard Miller, at home and reduced his dosage. The next day, he died of a massive stroke. Meanwhile, the patient who was drawn in the laboratory, Mr. Milner, was in his attorney's office filing a lawsuit.

Discussion

Phlebotomy is a highly detailed invasive procedure that can have serious consequences if it is performed incorrectly or beneath the standard of care for phlebotomy. Each phlebotomy procedure has the potential to injure, disable, and even end the life of the patient if the procedure is not performed according to the standards as established by the Clinical and Laboratory Standards Institute. Patients who are misidentified, such as the patient in this case, can receive incompatible blood, be over- or undermedicated, and generally mismanaged if they are treated based on laboratory test results other than their own. Patients who suffer injuries during the venipuncture can be permanently disabled or disfigured and spend the rest of their life in pain. Patients who pass out after venipuncture procedures can suffer fractures and paralysis due to the phlebotomist's inattentiveness.

In this case, the phlebotomist and her supervisor committed multiple errors. Each one alone is significant enough to have resulted in liability on behalf of the phlebotomist's employer. The first error was performed by the phlebotomist and/or the phlebotomist's employer who cleared her after only 3 hours of supervision. It was written in the facility's policy manual that new phlebotomists must undergo 40 hours of supervision before drawing specimens unsupervised. However, because the phlebotomist was cleared after only 3 hours, the supervisor violated facility policy and put patients to be drawn by this phlebotomist at risk. When managers don't adhere to facility policy, there is little defense when a patient is injured as a result of the deviation.

The phlebotomist in this case committed at least six errors. The first mistake was to ask the patient "Are you Howard Miller?" Perhaps the patient was hard of hearing; perhaps the phlebotomist spoke too quickly for him to discern the subtle difference between his real last name, "Milner," and the name the phlebotomist spoke, "Miller." Regardless of the reason, because the phlebotomist did not ask the patient to state his name, she was not able to realize that the registration clerk handed the patient the forms belonging to another patient. By coincidence, the paperwork she received in this case was for a patient who was also on heparin and who would be drawn later that day for the same test. This situation is not at all out of the realm of possibility in any healthcare facility.

Correct patient identification is the first and most vital step to a successful specimen collection procedure. According to the Clinical and Laboratory Standards Institute, proper outpatient identification consists of asking patients to give their full name, address, identification number, and/or birth date and to compare the information given with the information on the request form (1). Had this been properly performed according to the standards, the phlebotomist would likely have discovered the error.

The second error the phlebotomist committed was not surveying both arms for the presence of the medial vein. It is imperative that phlebotomists know the anatomy of the antecubital area, including the location of the veins, artery, and nerves that pass through the area. Because the most frequently injured nerve lies alongside, beneath, or even over the basilic vein, punctures to this vein should never be attempted unless all acceptable veins of both arms have been considered (1–5). Neglecting to consider alternative veins fails to reduce the risk of nerve injury to its greatest degree and can be argued in legal proceedings to be "operating beneath the standard of care." Although basilic veins are perfectly legitimate veins to access for phlebotomy purposes, they are not the safest for the patient. Therefore, phlebotomists must consider the other veins of the antecubital area (medial and cephalic) and make a professional judgment based on the risks of the procedure (1,3,4,7).

The third error committed was the needle relocation in the area known to be associated with nerve injuries. According to the Clinical and Laboratory Standards

Institute, "If the needle has penetrated too far into the vein, pull it back a bit. If it has not penetrated far enough, advance it farther into the vein. Rotate the needle half a turn. . . . Manipulation other than that recommended above is considered probing. Probing is not recommended."*

Probing is particularly risky in the area of the basilic vein. Therefore, any attempt to relocate the needle in this area puts the patient at great risk and should not be attempted (1,3,4). If an injury results and needle relocation can be demonstrated, it will be difficult to defend the technique in light of the standards.

The fourth error was the continued probing after the patient felt a shooting pain sensation. When a nerve is provoked, the patient feels a jolt of electricity shooting down the arm and sometimes up the arm to the shoulder. Because it cannot be suppressed, the phlebotomist is immediately aware that the nerve was involved. When presented with this reaction, the phlebotomist must end the venipuncture immediately before further damage ensues (3,4,7). Continued probing, as was done in this case study, can result in serious and permanent nerve damage and subject the phlebotomist and employer to liability. Therefore, attempts to relocate a needle after the patient feels excruciating, electric-like pain constitute perform- ance beneath the standard of care.

After needle withdrawal, a phlebotomist should apply pressure to the puncture site and assure that bleeding has stopped. Again, in this case, when the phle- botomist ended the venipuncture and allowed the patient to apply pressure on the puncture site, the phlebotomist handed over a responsibility that could lead to hematoma formation if the patient did not apply adequate force. Nerve injuries don't just occur when the needle strikes the nerve, but can also occur when the pressure of a hematoma weighs against the nerve (2,8). Allowing the patient to apply pressure may compromise and/or delay the sealing of the perforation made during venous access. Phlebotomists who allow patients to apply pressure must be assured that adequate pressure is being applied.

An even greater mistake was that the phlebotomist bandaged the site without checking to see if bleeding had stopped. According to the Clinical and Laboratory Standards Institute, the phlebotomist should "check that bleeding has ceased, ob- serve for hematoma, and apply an adhesive gauze or bandage over the venipunc- ture site" (1). This means assuring that not only the puncture through the skin has sealed, but that the puncture in the vein has sealed as well. Therefore, a two-point check is necessary to comply with the standards: (a) a visual observation for bleed- ing from the puncture through the skin; and (b) a visual observation for hematoma formation, which indicates that the vein has not sealed or that the artery may have been punctured. If the site is bandaged without performing both of these checks, the phlebotomist may be responsible for any bleeding that follows and the injuries that result from the bleeding. This is particularly important for patients who are on anticoagulant therapy.

The last critical error the phlebotomist committed turned an unfortunate injury into a catastrophe. By hastily leaving the patient's side, she failed to consider the

*Reproduced with permission, from CLSI/NCCLS publication H3-A5-Procedures for the Collection of Diagnostic Blood Specimens by Venipuncture; Approved Standard-Fifth Edition (ISBN 1-56238-515-1). Copies of the current edition may be obtained from the Clinical and Laboratory Standards Institute, 940 West Valley Road, Suite 1400, Wayne, Pennsylvania 19087-1898, USA.

potential all patients have: loss of consciousness after the venipuncture. Although infrequent, syncope is a known risk of the procedure. Therefore, all who collect blood specimens must be mindful of every patient's potential to pass out during or immediately after the phlebotomy procedure. Observation for the signs of an imminent loss of consciousness (e.g., pallor, perspiration, hyperventilation, anxiety, dizziness, etc.) and preparedness to react are important steps in a successful and safe phlebotomy procedure. Being prepared to react means never letting the patient out of sight while disposing of supplies, labeling tubes, or performing any other postpuncture activity. Should the phlebotomist lose sight of the patient, even momentarily, the phlebotomist may be liable for any injury that results while his/her attention was directed elsewhere. Patients should only be released from the care of a phlebotomist when the phlebotomist is reasonably certain that the patient will not lose consciousness. In the case described here, the patient was visibly at risk, yet the phlebotomist rushed out of the room prematurely.

After the patient was taken to the emergency room for evaluation and treatment, the real tragedy occurred. The real Mr. Howard Miller, who came to the same laboratory hours later that same day (with the proper paperwork), was tested and found to be properly medicated with heparin. However, when his physician received a call from the laboratory that he was overly medicated (based on Mr. Milner's improperly identified blood specimen), he was told to skip his next dose and cut subsequent doses in half. The next day, Mr. Miller, now undermedicated, developed a massive clot in his carotid artery, causing sudden death.

The other patient, Mr. Milner, had adverse reactions to the venipuncture procedure and decided to seek legal action against the facility. The patient believed that the phlebotomist was incompetent and sued the hospital for malpractice. Both the phlebotomist and her supervisor were deposed and endured harsh questioning from the patient's attorney who grilled them on their professional integrity during the deposition. It was an emotionally traumatic event for both of them. Both were subject to disciplinary action taken by the employer and documentation was entered in their employment files. Their employer settled out of court for an undisclosed amount.

The case study presented here is a composite of actual errors that phlebotomists have committed that have resulted in patient injury and lawsuits. Specimen collection errors are not only costly to the laboratory involved, they can be tragic for patients. Strict adherence to the standards for the procedure is the phlebotomists' only defense against liability. Those who are unfamiliar with the anatomy of the antecubital area should seek texts and educational resources to close the gaps in their understanding. Those who are unfamiliar with the Clinical and Laboratory Standards Institute's standards and the facility's procedure manual should conduct regular and thorough review of these documents. Managers who don't adhere to sound training and evaluation policies should be disciplined and/or educated so they may recommit to operating within the standards that exist in their facilities to fully protect their patients from injury and their employers from phlebotomy-related lawsuits.

REFERENCES

1. NCCLS. *Procedures for the collection of diagnostic blood specimens by venipuncture.* Approved Standard. H3-A5. Wayne, PA, 2003.
2. Horowitz S. Venipuncture-induced causalgia: anatomic relations of upper extremity superficial veins and nerves, and clinical considerations. *Transfusion* 2000;40:1036–1040.
3. Ernst D. Reduce your risk when you draw blood. *RN* 1999;62:65–66.
4. Ernst D. Phlebotomy meets the law. *Adv Admin Lab* 2001;10:27–36.
5. Ernst D. Phlebotomy on trial. *MLO* 1999;31:46–50.
6. Garza D, Becan-McBride K. *Phlebotomy handbook*, 6th ed. Upper Saddle River, NJ:Prentice Hall, 2002.
7. Masoorli S, Angeles T, Barbone. Danger points. How to prevent nerve injuries from venipuncture. *Nursing* 1998;September:35–39.

REVIEW QUESTIONS

1. Nerve injuries can occur by the excessive pressure exerted by hematomas or:
   a. when patients lose consciousness
   b. when the median cubital vein is punctured
   c. when the needle is inserted at a 30-degree angle or less
   d. when the needle comes in direct contact with the nerve
2. Asking patients to affirm their name as in "Are you John Smith?" is:
   a. acceptable only in stat situations
   b. never acceptable
   c. acceptable if the patient is unable to verbalize his/her name
   d. acceptable only if the patient has an identification bracelet attached to his or her wrist.
3. A reasonable and prudent phlebotomist knows that punctures to the basilic vein:
   a. pose the least risk of nerve or arterial involvement
   b. pose the greatest risk of nerve or arterial involvement
   c. pose moderate risk of nerve or arterial involvement
   d. pose no risk of nerve or arterial involvement
4. Which of the following structures of the antecubital area are most often injured during venipuncture procedures:
   a. nerves
   b. tendon
   c. bone
   d. muscle
5. A _____ vein should be considered in the absence of a visible or palpable medial vein.
   a. cephalic
   b. medial
   c. basilic
   d. hand
6. Due to the _____, punctures to the anterior aspect of the lower forearm should never be attempted:
   a. lack of nerves in the area
   b. presence of the basilic artery
   c. close proximity of nerves and tendons to the surface of the skin
   d. location of the radial artery
7. According to the Clinical and Laboratory Standards Institute and most textbooks, the proper angle of insertion for a venipuncture is:
   a. 15 degrees
   b. 30 degrees or less
   c. 30–45 degrees
   d. 45 degrees

8. Punctures outside of the antecubital area, the posterior aspect of the hand, and the lateral side of the wrist must be approached with a thorough knowledge of:
a. physiology
b. ergonomics
c. tort law
d. the anatomy of the structures under the skin in the selected area

Managing Exposures to Bloodborne Pathogens

8

Contributing Author: Ruth Carrico Ph.D., RN, CIC

Director, Infection Control and Infusion Services
University of Louisville Hospital
Louisville, Kentucky

INTRODUCTION

An accidental needlestick from a contaminated sharp is a terrifying experience affecting at least 385,000 healthcare workers in the United States every year (1). Those affected face agonizing decisions on their treatment and prophylaxis. In 2001, the *Morbidity and Mortality Weekly Report* published updated guidelines for management of the healthcare professional exposed to hepatitis B (HBV), hepatitis C (HCV), and HIV (2). This document provides an updated and well-defined process for evaluating exposures and recommending postexposure prophylaxis and forms the framework for exposure management. This chapter relies heavily on that document.

Exposures associated with blood collection procedures are not limited to accidental needlesticks. Therefore, this chapter will also address those exposures that can occur to nonintact skin and mucous membranes during blood collection, handling, and transportation and will stress the importance to all healthcare workers of taking personal responsibility for how to react in the event of an exposure. Since an effective exposure control plan is critical to protecting employees from acquiring bloodborne pathogens in the performance of their duties, a detailed section on exposure control plan development is included.

Because all healthcare workers should feel a sense of ownership in their facility's exposure control plan, readers are not only encouraged to be on the alert in their own workplace for unsafe practices, inadequate policies, and hazardous equipment, but to be well versed in what will be required of them should they be exposed to potentially infectious material.

After reading this chapter, the reader should be able to:

- List the keys to preexposure management
- Describe the actions that must be taken after an exposure
- List the body fluids capable of transmitting pathogens to the healthcare worker
- Evaluate an exposure based on the latest CDC recommendations
- Describe the treatment protocol for a high-titer exposure according to the CDC
- Discuss the elements of a comprehensive and functional exposure control plan

Because there are so many variables that determine the appropriate and necessary response to an accidental needlestick, cut, or splash, there is no single best course of action. Therefore, every healthcare professional must be aware of the treatment options as dictated by the variables unique to him/her and react accordingly. Those who manage specimen collection personnel must also be aware of the treatment options that apply to each individual under a variety of circumstances and work to ensure that their staff is prepared to act.

PREEXPOSURE MANAGEMENT

Understanding Bloodborne Pathogens

When determining the appropriate response to an exposure, the potential to acquire HBV, HCV, and HIV must be considered separately yet concurrently. Because these viruses are the most potentially infectious and pose the greatest risk to the exposed healthcare professional if acquired, an immediate evaluation of the source and severity of the exposure is paramount. The risk of transmission surrounding each exposure is dependent on factors unique to the circumstances and the individuals involved. Therefore, it is critical that the treatment given to those exposed takes into consideration all of the circumstances surrounding the exposure and reflects the current scientific consensus. Any exposure protocol that does not take into consideration the specifics of the injury puts the healthcare professional at risk of unnecessary procedures, treatments, and risks. The most effective exposure control plan is one that utilizes current knowledge on disease transmission and dictates highly specific actions based on individualized circumstances. In 1991, the Occupational Safety and Health Administration (OSHA) Bloodborne Pathogen Standard 29 CFR Part 1910.1030 included its list of body fluids representing a risk to healthcare workers. These body fluids are the following (3):

- Blood
- Semen
- Vaginal secretions

- Cerebrospinal fluid
- Synovial fluid
- Pleural fluid
- Pericardial fluid
- Peritoneal fluid
- Amniotic fluid
- Saliva in dental procedures
- Any body fluid that is visibly contaminated with blood
- All body fluids in situations where it is difficult or impossible to differentiate among those body fluids

Although it is important to understand which fluids represent the greatest risk, it is more important to understand which fluids represent the greatest *risk within the scope of an individual's practice.* The job responsibilities of any individual who provides patient care will place them at risk of exposure to some or all of those body fluids listed previously. Understanding one's own individual risk is an important component of prevention.

Prevention

Prevention is the most important aspect of an effective exposure control plan. When implementation of the plan gives high priority to preventative measures, the management of exposures is functioning at its highest level. According to OSHA, an exposure control plan must strive to reduce behaviors that lead to exposures (work practice controls) as well as implementing safer equipment, devices, supplies, and materials wherever possible (engineering controls) (3). Although healthcare facilities are required by OSHA to make personal protective equipment (PPE) readily available at no cost to the employee, healthcare professionals are not consistent in the use of this equipment. At Laval University in Quebec, a research group on behaviors in the health field determined that the application of Universal Precautions remains inadequate despite intensive education and intervention programs (4).

Although disease transmission to healthcare workers is serious and demands rigid adherence to prevention practices and postexposure policies, it's important to realize that an infection with a bloodborne pathogen is not automatic, even when the exposure is severe. However, healthcare workers should not allow this fact to lull them into a complacency that invites hazardous practices and neglectful behavior, leading to an exposure incident. Nor should it allow one to adopt a cavalier attitude toward the steps that must be taken after an exposure occurs. Immediate evaluation is critical to the prevention of disease transmission. Therefore, all healthcare facilities whose employees are subject to an ongoing risk of exposure should have an occupational health representative or infection control professional available to evaluate exposures around the clock.

Prevention of exposure is just as critical to an effective exposure control plan as the course of action to be taken in the event of an exposure. Safer equipment and devices alone will not reduce the risk of exposure to the staff to its greatest degree. Unsafe behaviors must also be eradicated. An in-depth discussion on preventive equipment and practices will be presented in Chapter 9.

Percutaneous injuries (e.g., a needlestick or cut with a sharp object) and contact of mucous membrane or nonintact skin (e.g., exposed skin that is chapped, abraded, or afflicted with dermatitis) with blood, tissue, or other body fluids that are potentially infectious are exposures that might place healthcare personnel at risk for HBV, HCV, or HIV infection (5,6). Accidental needlesticks are a common occupational risk when performing phlebotomy, but not the only one. Healthcare professionals responsible for centrifuging, processing, and/or transferring the serum or plasma to transfer tubes are subject to splashes into the eye, mucous membranes, or nonintact skin. Personal protection devices (i.e., face shields, splash guards, and protective eyewear) are available and provide essential protection for healthcare professionals.

The primary way to prevent transmission of HBV, HCV, and HIV in healthcare settings is to avoid blood exposures through use of barriers that prevent blood and body fluid contact. Preventing percutaneous injuries can also be accomplished by eliminating unnecessary needle use, implementing devices with safety features, using safe work practices when handling needles and other sharp devices, and safely disposing of sharps and blood-contaminated materials.

Preexposure Immunizations

The rate of occupationally acquired hepatitis dropped 90% with the advent of immunization programs against HBV in the 1980s. Since 1991, OSHA's Bloodborne Pathogen Standard has required healthcare facilities to offer immunizations to at-risk employees as a preventive measure (3). The immunization consists of a series of three injections administered over 6 months. The healthcare professional should be tested for antibody production 30 to 60 days after the final injection. The series should be repeated if antibodies are not present in numbers sufficient to indicate immunity. If antibodies are still not present after the second series, the healthcare professional should be evaluated to determine if he/she is a chronic carrier of the virus (2,7). If a chronic carrier status is confirmed, the healthcare professional should be counseled in-depth about the risks of transmitting the virus during patient care and about appropriate prevention strategies. The employee's manager should evaluate the work responsibilities of the chronic carrier to ensure patient safety. If testing reveals that a chronic carrier state does not exist, the person can be considered a nonconverter, i.e., his/her body will not produce antibodies to the virus and immunity may be unattainable. For these individuals, preventing HBV exposure and rapidly reporting exposure situations is of paramount importance.

Currently, there are no preventive vaccines recommended for HCV or HIV (2,7). HCV is transmitted by blood and body fluids and is the most common chronic bloodborne infection in the United States. HIV is estimated to have infected more than 60 million people worldwide with almost 1 million infected persons living in the United States (8).

Research estimates that the average risk for HIV transmission after a percutaneous exposure to HIV-infected blood is approximately 0.3% (9,10). Occupational transmission of HIV from patients to healthcare professionals may occur through nonintact skin such as cuts, abrasions, and punctures (percutaneous), or, less frequently, through mucous membranes (mucocutaneous). For both of these diseases, the best protection involves the use of personal protective equipment when processing blood and body fluids and caution when handling needles and body fluids.

All healthcare personnel should be aware of these key concepts about bloodborne pathogens:

- Infection with a bloodborne pathogen is not automatic following even the most severe exposures
- Prevention strategies are an important component of a safety program for healthcare personnel
- An occupational health department representative or an alternative should be available 24 hours a day, 7 days a week in all facilities that present an ongoing risk of exposure to their employees
- Although it is essential that healthcare personnel understand methods of transmission, exposure prevention strategies, and workplace practices that put them at risk, knowing how to react is the next line of defense.

POSTEXPOSURE MANAGEMENT

Any exposure to blood or other potentially infectious material should be considered a medical emergency. When exposed, the healthcare worker must immediately engage the exposure control plan by (1) conducting immediate wound (or mucous membrane) care, (2) evaluating the exposure to determine the risk of disease transmission, and (3) investigating the source patient of the contaminating fluid. In some situations, preventive medications should be administered immediately, ideally within hours of the exposure. Should the exposure be considered low risk, the decision to administer antiretroviral drugs is difficult in light of their association with serious and debilitating side effects. Therefore, immediate access to a skilled employee health provider to evaluate the severity and risk factors of an exposure and manage an appropriate response is the cornerstone of an effective exposure management program. This mechanism requires around-the-clock, year-round access to the process.

Actions that should be taken after an exposure include the following:

- Care of the exposure site (wound or mucous membrane)
- Evaluation of the exposure to determine risk, necessity for source testing and for postexposure prophylactic administration

- Testing and counseling for the source patient
- Follow-up care and counseling for the healthcare professional

Percutaneous Wound Care

Accidental exposure to the tissue by a puncture with a contaminated needle, a cut by broken glass contaminated with body fluids, or body fluids coming into contact with nonintact skin demands immediate attention. These exposures are associated with the highest risk of acquiring HIV, HBV, and HCV infection (seroconversion) if present in the fluid. Immediately upon injury, the site should be thoroughly washed and assessed by a clinician. The care provided to the site depends on the nature of the exposure. Regardless of whether the exposure involves a wound, nonintact skin, or contact with a mucous membrane, the healthcare worker must wash and disinfect the site immediately.

Immediate wound care includes the following for cuts and needlesticks:

- Wash the site with soap and water taking care to remove any foreign object(s) that may also be in the wound
- There is no need for scrubbing, squeezing, or use of chemicals on the wound

For mucous membrane exposures, immediate wound care includes the following:

- Gently irrigate with tap water, sterile saline, or sterile water for several minutes taking care to remove any foreign objects or debris
- Exposures involving the eye should include gentle, continuous, and thorough irrigation as from an eyewash station
- Contact lenses should be removed as soon as possible and disinfected according to the manufacturer's recommendation or, if disposable, the lenses should be discarded

Exposure Evaluation

After an exposure, the appropriate response must consider the potential for the injured healthcare worker to acquire HBV, HCV, and HIV concurrently. Once each risk is assessed, each will require its own response based on a multitude of variables unique to the exposure. It is important to realize that not all exposures lead to a reasonable risk of acquiring a bloodborne pathogen. For example, other than immediate wound care, an accidental needlestick with a needle used during an unsuccessful venipuncture attempt may not require further action.

The time just after an injury is a time of intense anxiety for the injured. If it is also a time of anxiety for the individual responsible for implementing the facility's postexposure protocol, then the risk of disease transmission increases. Likewise, the risk of inappropriately administering antiretrovirals increases as well. It is just as important to know when testing and treatment is necessary as to know when it is not. To evaluate the severity of an exposure, it is crucial to establish whether or not an exchange of blood could have occurred. Some factors to consider include:

- The severity of the exposure
- The route of entry
- The amount of blood involved in the exposure
- The epidemiologic likelihood that the healthcare professional was exposed to HBV, HCV, or HIV

The risk of acquiring a bloodborne pathogen from a needle used in an intramuscular (IM) injection is significantly less than that from a needle used in blood collection (2). Therefore, the treatment for an accidental needlestick from a needle that had not punctured a vein may not be the same as for that from a needle that had accessed a vein. The individual sustaining the injury has the most crucial information needed to assess the severity of the exposure. However, in times of stress and anxiety, the individual may not be thinking clearly enough or rationally enough to put a plan into effect. It is paramount, therefore, that someone be immediately available to ask the right questions and implement the appropriate events to minimize the potential for disease transmission and the inappropriate use of antiretroviral medications. The most appropriate healthcare professional to implement the appropriate response is the infection control or occupational health nurse and/or a trained infectious diseases physician. Once it has been determined that the accident has put the healthcare professional at risk, a systematic approach to treatment is best conducted by considering the risk of acquiring each infection separately.

 Tips from the Trenches: It should not be assumed that the treatment for an accidental needlestick from a needle that had not yet punctured a vein is the same as for that from a needle that had accessed a vein.

Postexposure Prophylaxis

Hepatitis B

If not immunized, the risk associated with accidental needlestick inoculation of HBV-infected blood varies between 5% and 35%. Viral transmission is dependent on the source's hepatitis B e-antigen (HBeAg) status and, if infected, the viral titer (5,11,12). Transmission can be considered unlikely if records or knowledge exist that the healthcare professional has been successfully immunized. Under current recommendations, retesting is not necessary and no treatment is required (2).

However, the source patient should be tested for the presence of the hepatitis B surface antigen (HBsAg) if the exposed healthcare worker has not been immunized with the hepatitis B vaccine or if the immune status is not known. If the patient tests positive, hepatitis B-specific immune globulin

(HBIG) should be given intramuscularly at a dose of 0.06 mL/kg body weight, ideally within 24 hours of the exposure but no later than 7 days. HBIG is given in a larger muscle (e.g., gluteus) due to the volume administered. A second dose may be indicated in 30 days. HBIG, however, is only effective for 70% to 85% of those to whom it is administered (13). In addition to HBIG, the hepatitis B vaccine should be initiated at this time if the healthcare professional has not yet received the series of immunizations. If the series is incomplete, the dose should be administered intramuscularly at the same time as the HBIG but using a different site. (The hepatitis B vaccine is always given in the deltoid muscle using a needle of sufficient length to ensure that the dose is administered intramuscularly.)

If the source patient tests negative for the HbsAg, it indicates that the patient probably does not harbor the hepatitis B virus and is incapable of transmitting it. Therefore, no prophylaxis is generally indicated for exposed healthcare personnel. Conceivably, the patient could be in the early stage of a hepatitis B infection that is not yet detectable by laboratory measurements. Exposure to the blood of a patient in this early stage is considered low-risk and no treatment is indicated.

If the exposed healthcare worker is undergoing the series of hepatitis B immunizations at the time of the exposure, consideration may be given to baseline testing to determine if the immunizations have been successful. This may prevent the unnecessary administration of HBIG. Despite the identification of antibodies, any remaining dose(s) of the vaccine should continue as scheduled. If the source of the exposure is unknown or cannot be determined (e.g., exposure to one of many needles protruding from a sharps container), the exposure must generally be treated as if it were from a patient who has HBV. The proper protocol for protecting an exposed healthcare worker from acquiring hepatitis B, therefore, is dependent on the worker's immune status. Table 8.1 summarizes recommendations for prophylaxis after percutaneous, mucosal, or nonintact skin exposure to blood according to the HBsAg status of the exposure source and the vaccination and vaccine-response status of the exposed person (2).

Hepatitis C

HCV is not transmitted efficiently through occupational exposures to blood. Healthcare professionals who are exposed to infected blood through needlestick injuries may acquire HCV infection, but the magnitude of risk (approximately 1.8%) is less than that associated with HBV exposure. One epidemiologic study indicated that transmission occurred only from hollow-bore needles compared with other sharps (14). Transmission rarely occurs from mucous membrane exposures to blood, and more rarely has been documented from nonintact skin exposures to blood (15).

For persons exposed to an HCV-negative source, no testing needs to be done on the exposed healthcare professional. For persons exposed to an HCV-positive source, testing for the HCV antibody (anti-HCV) by immunoassay and ALT activity is recommended at baseline and 4 to 6 months after the

TABLE 8.1 ■ Recommended Postexposure Prophylaxis for Exposure to Hepatitis B Virus (b)

Vaccination and Antibody Response Status of Exposed Healthcare Personnel*	Treatment		
	Source HBsAg[†] Positive	Source HBsAg[†] Negative	Source Unknown or Not Available for Testing
Unvaccinated	HBIG[§] × 1 and initiate hepatitis B vaccine series	Initiate hepatitis B vaccine series	Initiate hepatitis B vaccine series
Previously vaccinated			
Known responder[¶]	No treatment	No treatment	No treatment
Known nonresponder**	HBIG × 1 and initiate revaccination or HBIG × 2*[†]	No treatment	If known high-risk source, treat as if source were HBsAg positive
Antibody response unknown	Test exposed person for anti-HBs[§§]: 1. If adequate,[¶] no treatment is necessary 2. If inadequate,** HBIG × 1 and vaccine booster	No treatment	Test exposed person for anti-HBs: 1. If adequate, no treatment is necessary 2. If inadequate, administer vaccine booster and recheck titer in 1–2 months

*Persons who have previously been infected with HBV are immune to reinfection and do not require postexposure prophylaxis.
[†]Hepatitis B surface antigen.
[§]Hepatitis B immune globulin; dose in 0.06 mL/kg intramuscularly.
[¶]A responder is a person with adequate levels of serum antibody to HBsAg (i.e., anti-HBS ≥10 mIU/mL).
**A nonresponder is a person with inadequate response to vaccination (i.e., serum anti-HBS <10 mIU/mL).
[††]The option of giving 1 dose of HBIG and reinitiating the vaccine series is preferred for nonresponders who have not completed a second 3-dose vaccine series. For persons who previously completed a second vaccine series but failed to respond, two doses of HBIG are preferred.
[§§]Antibody to HBsAg.

exposure to detect infection; testing for HCV-RNA may be performed 4 to 6 weeks after exposure if earlier detection of infection is desired (2). No clinical trials have been conducted to assess postexposure use of antiviral agents (e.g., interferon with or without ribavirin) to prevent HCV infection, and antivirals are not FDA-approved for this application. Available data suggest that an established infection might need to be present before interferon can be an effective treatment (2,16).

Because there is currently no postexposure prophylaxis for HCV, the intent of recommendations for postexposure management is to achieve early identification of chronic disease and, if present, refer the individual for evaluation of treatment options. In addition, no guidelines exist for administration of therapy during the acute phase of HCV infection. However, limited data indicate that antiviral therapy might be beneficial when started early in the course of HCV infection. When HCV infection is identified early, the exposed person should be referred to a specialist for medical management. Avoidance of exposure to blood, primarily through percutaneous injury, is the only currently available strategy for preventing HCV infection (2).

HIV

Although the transmission of HIV from an accidental needlestick is usually the greatest concern to the exposed, it poses the least likelihood of transmission (0.3%) of the viruses discussed (5,11,12). Groups of workers at risk for acquiring HIV infection occupationally are healthcare personnel and other workers in contact with blood or other body fluids who sustain accidental percutaneous or mucosal inoculations with HIV-infected material. The magnitude of risk depends on the severity of exposure, but on the average, is about 0.3% after percutaneous injury. The risk of infection following mucosal exposures is estimated to be lower (approximately 0.09%). In the absence of direct exposure, healthcare personnel are not at occupational risk for HIV infection. In the United States, through December 2002, 57 healthcare professionals were documented as having seroconverted to HIV following occupational exposures (17). In addition, 139 other cases of HIV infection or AIDS have occurred among healthcare personnel who have not reported other risk factors for HIV infection and who report a history of occupational exposure to blood, body fluids, or HIV-infected laboratory material, but for whom seroconversion after exposure was not documented. The number of these workers who acquired their infection through occupational exposures is unknown.

However, because it is more devastating to acquire than either hepatitis B or C, aggressive measures must be considered immediately after a blood exposure has occurred—ideally within hours of the event (2). Because of the emotional impact that exposure to this virus presents, healthcare professionals must be educated before an exposure occurs as to the appropriate actions they will have to take. Familiarity with the process is critical.

The actions that exposed healthcare personnel should take depend on a number of variables. An awareness of the variables greatly simplifies the process during the anxiety that surrounds most accidental exposures. When it has been determined that the source should be tested for HIV, the patient's blood that will be tested for HIV should be drawn into a tube that allows clotting (i.e., plain, nonadditive tube or gel tube with clot activator) and immediately transported to the laboratory. Simultaneously, tubes can be filled for HBV and HCV testing as required. Rapid HIV tests that provide results within minutes are available. The laboratory should be consulted about the type of rapid HIV test it performs so that the specimen can be collected properly.

Some states require the patient's "informed consent" before the test can be performed. However, laws outlining the requirements for obtaining informed consent from the source patient vary from state to state. If consent is required, an individual other than the exposed employee should obtain it. When informed consent is not possible, the patient's physician should be notified and requested to facilitate testing. Occasionally, the healthcare facility's legal counsel may need to address informed consent issues in concert with the executive staff and/or the facility's risk manager. Preplanning for potential obstacles is essential to a functional exposure control plan.

 Tips from the Trenches: *All healthcare personnel should project themselves into their facility's exposure control plan before it becomes necessary to assure that (1) the plan itself is intact, and (2) the steps that will become necessary in the event of an exposure will be familiar.*

The facility's postexposure plan must be implemented in every exposure to HIV-positive blood to prevent disease transmission. A facility's plan must reflect those variables in risk, staffing structure, and accessibility to the facility's chemoprophylactic agents. It is important that the plan can be initiated immediately and followed in the event of an exposure regardless of the time of the exposure or the location of the employee.

The pharmacologic preventative that a facility adopts for use after a qualifying exposure to HIV is referred to as the facility's postexposure prophylaxis (PEP). For HIV, PEP therapy is aggressive, lengthy (usually 4 weeks), and subjects those who receive it to serious and potentially debilitating side effects. Therefore, its administration must be justified.

Workers sustaining accidental parenteral exposures to HIV should be counseled to undergo baseline and follow-up testing for 6 months after exposure (e.g., 6 weeks, 3 months, and 6 months) to diagnose infection. Since 1996, the U.S. Public Health Service has recommended postexposure chemoprophylaxis (PEP) with antiretroviral agents after certain exposures to HIV-infected sources that pose a risk of infection transmission, such as needlesticks, mucous membrane, and nonintact skin exposures (Tables 8.2 and 8.3) (2). Most HIV exposures will warrant a two-drug regimen using two nucleoside analogues (e.g., zidovudine and lamivudine [3TC]; or 3TC and stavudine [d4T]; or d4T and didanosine [ddI]). The addition of a third drug should be considered for exposures that pose an increased risk for transmission. Updated guidelines that include additional antiretrovirals, such as boosted protease inhibitors, for HIV PEP are being developed. Selection of the PEP regimen should take into consideration the comparative risk represented by the exposure and information about the exposure source, including history of and response to antiretroviral therapy based on clinical response, CD4+ T-cell counts, viral load measurements, and current disease stage. Data from animal models of prophylaxis with these agents suggest that antiviral activity is diminished when treatment is delayed for more than 24 hours. For this reason, immediate reporting and access to PEP are recommended.

In addition to follow-up serologic testing, monitoring for PEP toxicity is needed if PEP is taken. A complete blood count as well as renal and hepatic profiles should be done at baseline and 2 weeks after starting PEP. If the PEP regimen includes a protease inhibitor, the exposed person also should be monitored for hypoglycemia, crystalluria, hematuria, hemolytic anemia, and hepatitis. The PEP regimen should be discontinued or modified and expert consultation obtained if PEP toxicity develops.

TABLE 8.2 ■ Recommended HIV Postexposure Prophylaxis for Percutaneous Injuries (5)

Exposure Type	Infection Status of Source				
	HIV Positive, Class 1*	HIV Positive, Class 2*	Known Source, Unknown HIV Status†	Unknown Source§	HIV Negative
Less severe¶	Recommend basic 2-drug PEP	Recommend expanded 3-drug PEP	Generally, no PEP warranted; however, consider basic 2-drug PEP** for source with HIV risk factors††	Generally, no PEP warranted; however, consider basic 2-drug PEP** in settings where exposure to HIV-infected persons is likely	No PEP warranted
More severe§§	Recommend expanded 3-drug PEP	Recommend expanded 3-drug PEP	Generally, no PEP warranted; however, consider basic 2-drug PEP** for source with HIV risk factors††	Generally, no PEP warranted; however, consider basic 2-drug PEP** in settings where exposure to HIV-infected persons is likely	No PEP warranted

*HIV positive, Class 1—asymptomatic HIV infection or known low viral load (e.g., <1,500 RNA copies/mL). HIV positive, Class 2—symptomatic HIV infection, AIDS, acute seroconversion, or known high viral load. If drug resistance is a concern, obtain expert consultation. Initiation of postexposure prophylaxis (PEP) should not be delayed pending expert consultation, and, because expert consultation alone cannot substitute for face-to-face counseling, resources should be available to provide immediate evaluation and follow-up care for all exposures.

†Source of unknown HIV status (e.g., deceased source person with no samples available for HIV testing).

§Unknown source (e.g., a needle from a sharps disposal container).

¶Less severe (e.g., solid needle and superficial injury).

**The designation, "consider PEP," indicates that PEP is optional and should be based on an individualized decision between the exposed person and the treating clinician.

††If PEP is offered and taken, and the source is later determined to be HIV negative, PEP should be discontinued.

§§More severe (e.g., large-bore hollow needle, deep puncture, visible blood on device, or needle used in patient's artery or vein).

TABLE 8.3 ■ Recommended HIV Postexposure Prophylaxis for Mucous Membrane Exposures and Nonintact Skin* Exposures (5)

Exposure Type	HIV Positive, Class 1*	HIV Positive, Class 2†	Infection Status of Source Source Known, Unknown HIV Status§	Unknown Source¶	HIV Negative
Small volume**	Consider basic 2-drug PEP††	Recommend basic 2-drug PEP	Generally, no PEP warranted; however, consider basic 2-drug PEP†† for source with HIV risk factors§§	Generally, no PEP warranted; however, consider basic 2-drug PEP†† in settings where exposure to HIV-infected persons is likely	No PEP warranted
Large volume¶¶	Recommend basic 2-drug PEP	Recommend expanded 3-drug PEP	Generally, no PEP warranted; however, consider basic 2-drug PEP†† for source with HIV risk factors§§	Generally, no PEP warranted; however, consider basic 2-drug PEP†† in settings where exposure to HIV-infected persons is likely	No PEP warranted

*For skin exposures, follow-up is indicated only if there is evidence of compromised skin integrity (e.g., dermatitis, abrasion, or open wound).

†HIV Positive, Class 1—asymptomatic HIV infection or known low viral load (e.g., <1,500 RNA copies/mL). HIV Positive, Class 2—symptomatic HIV infection, AIDS, acute seroconversion, or known high viral load. If drug resistance is a concern, obtain expert consultation. Initiation of postexposure prophylaxis (PEP) should be available to provide immediate evaluation and follow-up care for all exposures.

§Source of unknown HIV status (e.g., deceased source person with no samples available for HIV testing).

¶Unknown source (e.g., splash from inappropriately disposed blood).

**Small volume (i.e., a few drops).

††The designation, "consider PEP," indicates that PEP is optional and should be based on an individualized decision between the exposed person and the treating clinician.

§§If PEP is offered and taken, and the source is later determined to be HIV negative, PEP should be discontinued.

¶¶Large volume (i.e., major blood splash).

Because occupational exposure to HIV can be a frightening experience, consultation with clinicians knowledgeable about HIV transmission risks who can provide supportive counseling to the worker is essential during the follow-up interval. The Centers for Disease Control (CDC) recommends that occupationally exposed workers refrain from unsafe sexual practices, pregnancy, breastfeeding, and blood and organ donation for 6 months after exposure.

Because of the urgency of intervention following an HIV-positive exposure, an exposure control plan must be so well established that it is able to evaluate candidacy and administer appropriate PEP on short notice, 24 hours a day, 7 days a week. A facility with an exposure control plan unable to meet this objective fails to meet the basic intent of the plan and, therefore, fails to protect its work force. Table 8.2 provides recommendations for HIV prophylaxis for percutaneous injury and Table 8.3 provides recommendations for HIV postexposure prophylaxis for mucous membrane and nonintact skin exposures based on the most current CDC recommendations.

Although each facility must ultimately establish its own criteria for PEP administration based on established guidelines such as the CDC recommendations, some general considerations apply:

- The healthcare professional must have been exposed to blood from a known HIV-positive patient or to body fluid containing visible blood from a known HIV-positive patient

or

- The healthcare professional must have been exposed to blood or body fluid containing visible blood from an individual who is at a high risk of being infected with HIV, but whose status is unknown at the time of exposure

or

- The healthcare professional has been exposed to a source of undetermined origin

If the source is unknown, additional factors to consider include the prevalence of HIV in the community and patient population. Unless the patient's HIV status can be determined within hours of the exposure, healthcare professionals should be prepared to make a decision on whether or not to receive the facility's PEP as a preventive measure. If they decide to begin the facility's PEP therapy and the patient later tests negative, the PEP can be discontinued. If they decide not to begin PEP therapy and the patient later tests positive, they may have compromised their defense against acquiring the virus. Because of the side effects of the current PEP therapies, however, those exposed to blood of undetermined risk must weigh the consequences of action and inaction carefully and make a personal decision whether or not to receive the facility's PEP.

Postexposure Testing and Counseling

Testing the Employee

Postexposure testing for hepatitis B involves testing the exposed employee for HBsAg at the time of exposure and again after 6 months if the healthcare professional is nonimmune after attempted immunization or has never been immunized, and

■ The source is antigen-positive for HBV

or

■ The source is unknown

If the healthcare professional experiences symptoms consistent with acute retroviral syndrome or hepatitis regardless of the interval since exposure, interim testing may be performed (Box 8.1).

For HCV, no postexposure immunization is available. However, testing should be done on the exposed healthcare professional at the time of the exposure and after 6 months if one of the following conditions exist:

■ The source is positive for anti-HCV

or

■ The source is unknown

Again, interim testing may be performed if the individual experiences symptoms consistent with acute retroviral syndrome or hepatitis regardless of the interval since exposure.

For HIV, antibody testing should be performed at the time of the exposure (baseline), then 6 weeks, 12 weeks, and 6 months after the exposure if one of the following conditions exists:

■ The source is positive for HIV

or

■ The source is unknown

BOX 8.1   Symptoms of Acute Retroviral Syndrome

Exposed healthcare workers should also be counseled regarding the importance of seeking medical evaluation for any acute illness that occurs during the follow-up period. Exhibiting the following symptoms may indicate acute seroconversion and the individual healthcare professional should be evaluated immediately by a skilled clinician. Acute retroviral syndrome is characterized by:

■ Fever	■ Fatigue
■ Rash	■ Malaise
■ Myalgia	■ Lymphadenopathy

As with hepatitis B and C, interim testing may be performed if the health-care professional experiences symptoms consistent with acute retroviral syndrome regardless of the interval since exposure. Antiretrovirals should be administered as soon as possible after a qualifying exposure and continued for 4 weeks until the exposure has been proved to be negligible.

Counseling the Employee

In the critical time following an exposure, the injured healthcare professional may be incapable of making rational decisions. Therefore, it is of paramount importance that facilities be prepared to counsel healthcare personnel exposed to potentially infectious blood so that informed, levelheaded decisions can lead to appropriate action. In addition, there is comfort in being counseled by clinicians experienced in dealing with occupational exposures and knowledgeable of the facility's exposure control plan. Counseling should include:

- Immediate therapy options indicated by the nature of the exposure
- Information on follow-up testing
- Information about the possibility of transmitting any viruses acquired from the exposure to family, patients, and other contacts
- Ways to prevent such secondary transmissions
- The implications of current or future pregnancies if appropriate
- Symptoms of virus transmission
- Side effects of the facility's prescribed PEP if administered

Because the need for counseling is urgent and significant, facilities should make such services available 24 hours a day. The CDC recommends that healthcare professionals with occupational exposure receive follow-up counseling, appropriate testing, and medical evaluation regardless of whether or not the facility's PEP was administered.

Healthcare personnel who acquire HBV, HCV, or HIV remain potentially infectious to others. Those exposed should be advised to use measures to prevent secondary transmission until it has been established that they have not acquired a transmissible virus. These measures include the following:

- Sexual abstinence or use of condoms
- Defer pregnancy
- Refrain from donating blood, plasma, organs, tissue, or semen
- Discontinue breast-feeding, especially following high-risk exposures
- Strict adherence to universal precautions
- Promptly reporting incidences in which healthcare professionals have put patients at risk through exposure to their blood or other potentially infectious fluids

When the prescribed PEP is administered, the exposed healthcare worker must receive counseling on food and drug interactions, side effects, adherence to time and dosage regimens, and the body's need for increased fluid intake. Side effects that may require immediate attention include: back or abdominal pain, pain on urination, blood in urine, or symptoms of hyperglycemia. Pregnant recipients require special attention since both mother and baby may be directly affected. Finally, it is important for the exposed individual to adhere to the schedule for follow-up blood work. These tests may be ordered weekly and depend on the medication(s) included in the PEP, preexisting medical history of the exposed healthcare professional, and other factors.

Especially important is that the exposed individual obtains emotional support during the 6-month period immediately following an exposure, especially in the event of a high-risk exposure. All counseling and follow-up care should be done in an environment that maintains confidentiality and allows sufficient time to answer questions and address concerns.

Testing and Counseling the Source Patient

If investigation of the exposure leads to the conclusion that a high-risk exposure has occurred (see Tables 8.2 and 8.3), then testing of the source, if it can be determined, must include HCV and HIV using the CDC recommendations (2). If the healthcare worker's HBV immunization records cannot be referenced, HBV testing is necessary. The patient from whom the contaminated sharp originated should be counseled with regard to his or her test results. Test results must be communicated by a clinician skilled in counseling—especially if the patient tested positive—with privacy and in an atmosphere that minimizes distractions. These details should be included in the facility's exposure management plan. Generally, it is the responsibility of the ordering clinician to share the test results with the source patient.

SUMMARY OF EXPOSURE PROTOCOL

Hepatitis B

- Prophylactic treatment and source testing is not indicated if the healthcare professional has been previously immunized with the hepatitis B vaccine and the immunization has been proved to be successful. Transmission is unlikely to occur.
- If the healthcare professional has not been immunized or the success of immunization cannot be determined, the source patient (if known) should be tested for the presence of HBsAg. If the patient tests positive, the healthcare professional should receive HBIG at a dose of 0.06 mL/kg body weight IM within 48 hours (preferably, but no longer than within 7 days) of the exposure. Treatment should be repeated in 30 days. In addition, the series of hepatitis B immunizations should be initiated. If the patient tests negative, no immunization or treatment for the prevention of HBV transmission is indicated.

- Healthcare professionals currently undergoing the immunization series should be tested for their immune status (HBsAb) and treated accordingly.
- If the source of the exposure cannot be identified and the healthcare professional tests negative (nonimmune) or the immune status cannot be determined, the exposed employee should begin hepatitis B immunizations.

Hepatitis C

- Test the patient source (if known) for the hepatitis C antibody (anti-HCV). If positive, monitor the exposed healthcare worker for symptoms of hepatitis.
- Test the exposed individual for baseline anti-HCV at the time of the exposure and again after 6 months. Monitor for symptoms of hepatitis.

HIV

Because of the complexity of the protocol for reacting to a potential HIV exposure, refer to Tables 8.2 and 8.3, the recommended CDC post-HIV exposure prophylaxis.

ELEMENTS OF A COMPREHENSIVE AND FUNCTIONAL EXPOSURE CONTROL PLAN

There are many components of an exposure control plan that are necessary to guarantee that healthcare personnel exposed to bloodborne pathogens receive the most timely, confidential, and effective care and treatment to prevent disease transmission. Employees must sense that the exposure control plan and the personnel responsible for implementing it have a passionate concern for their well-being. Such concern is directly proportional to the complexity of the facility's plan. A broad range of contingencies and obstacles must be considered for the plan to be fully functional, and the plan must be universally applicable at all times to all employees regardless of the personnel on duty. The following checklist may be helpful to assess the functionality of your facility's plan. Deficiencies should be addressed before the need arises. The plan should:

- Accommodate on-site as well as off-site work-related injuries
- Ensure that mechanisms are in place to accomplish rapid and immediate HIV testing. This includes test ordering, specimen collection, specimen transportation, billing, and result reporting
- Clearly define the steps that injured healthcare personnel should take to ensure the best and most appropriate treatment of their exposure
- Include the protocol necessary to collect and test the patient's blood for bloodborne pathogens. This should include the location of consent

forms and the circumstances under which consent is not necessary. It should also define who should collect the blood, how the blood should be collected, and where the blood should be sent for testing

- Reflect the current consensus on preventive therapies when establishing its PEP and be reviewed and revised on a regular basis
- Identify the criteria for administration of the PEP and detail those conditions in which PEP is not indicated
- Guarantee that the PEP is not only available, but also accessible, 24 hours a day, 7 days a week, 365 days a year
- Arrange for the PEP prescriptions to be written by physicians and filled at locations that preserve the healthcare professional's confidentiality if it becomes an issue
- Guarantee that HBIG is available for administration within 48 hours after any exposure.
- Not require costly medications to be paid for by the healthcare worker regardless of reimbursement
- Have a mechanism in place so that an occupational health professional is immediately available to implement the plan, resolve problems, and counsel the injured

Being alert for weaknesses and potential failures in the plan before an injury occurs requires the scrutiny of many individuals dedicated to preventing disease transmission. Recruiting the assistance of nonadministrative personnel helps to give employees a sense of ownership in the plan. One key component of establishing and maintaining an effective exposure control plan is to test its effectiveness periodically.

Assessing Effectiveness

Managers and employers of healthcare personnel have a legal and moral obligation to their employees to provide a safe working environment that minimizes risk of injuries that can be reasonably anticipated during the performance of their duties. This includes the ability to respond promptly, effectively, and completely to injuries sustained and illnesses acquired on the job. A comprehensive and functional exposure control plan demonstrates the fulfillment of this obligation.

Not all comprehensive plans are fully functional and not all functional plans are comprehensive. It is imperative that those who collect and/or handle blood specimens scrutinize their employer's plan to make sure it will protect them against acquiring a bloodborne pathogen. Because the activities of each employee can vary significantly, those who develop and implement an exposure control plan in their facility may not be able to anticipate the risk for all employees or prepare for all contingencies. For this reason, it is critical that all employees become familiar with the plan and take the initiative to assess the plan's effectiveness in light of their daily routine and risk factors.

Tips from the Trenches: *A comprehensive and functional exposure control plan demonstrates the fulfillment of an employer's obligation to provide a safe working environment that minimizes risk of exposure to blood or other potentially infectious materials that can be reasonably anticipated during the performance of the duties of their employees.*

To test the functionality of an existing exposure control plan, walk through the steps you would take if you are exposed to blood through an accidental needlestick or through nonintact skin or mucous membrane contact regardless of the day or time. The following list of questions should be asked:

- Whom should I notify when I have an accidental needlestick or other percutaneous injury?
- Where should I go for immediate care?
- Are they prepared to treat me immediately and administer the appropriate PEP within 2 hours of my exposure, if necessary?
- Who will administer the PEP if I need it?
- If the PEP is not on hand, is there a mechanism in place for obtaining it immediately 24 hours a day, 365 days a year?
- What forms am I supposed to fill out?
- Will those forms be available when I need them?
- Is there an eyewash station or bottle in the area where I process specimens?
- Where should I go for baseline lab work?
- What baseline lab work should be drawn and what tubes are required?
- What physician will order the lab work?
- Will I be expected to pay for the lab work?
- Who will pay for the PEP if I need it?
- If I am to be reimbursed for the lab work or PEP, what if I don't have enough money to pay for it up-front?
- Can I go to an off-site laboratory to protect my confidentiality?
- If so, how will the laboratory be paid?
- If the physician receives the results, how and when will I be notified?
- Who else will see my lab results?
- Who will determine if I need the PEP?
- How do I assess the risk of the exposure?
- What tests should be ordered and performed on the source patient's blood?
- If the source patient's blood is already available in the laboratory, can it be used to perform source testing?
- What tubes should be drawn on the source patient for postexposure testing?
- What tubes should be drawn from me for postexposure testing?
- Do I need the patient's permission to draw and test for HIV? Hepatitis?
- What if the patient refuses to be tested?

- Where will the patient's testing be performed?
- Does the testing lab have a mechanism in place for testing and reporting postexposure cases within hours?
- If testing is done off-site, how does the specimen reach the lab?
- Who will pay for the patient's testing?
- What is my immune status for hepatitis?
- Are contingencies in place if I stick myself on third shift, a weekend, or during a holiday?
- When was the plan last tested?
- What if the emergency department is too busy to attend to my injury and treatment in a timely manner?
- Should I still take the PEP if I am pregnant?
- What are the risks of transmitting an acquired virus to my spouse? My family?

There are a multitude of details that have to be considered and accommodated in a functional and comprehensive exposure control plan. Not all facilities have the resources to put such a plan in place. As healthcare professionals who may have to rely on their facility's existing plan to protect them with the most up-to-date concepts in postexposure treatment, it is imperative that deficiencies be identified and eliminated through a cooperative effort before the plan fails to protect an injured employee. Healthcare personnel should evaluate the ability of their facility's exposure control plan to respond to a variety of realistic circumstances and conditions before they are put to the test. Any gaps or inadequacies should be communicated and cooperatively resolved. Healthcare professionals without administrative responsibilities can be instrumental in improving existing mechanisms and should welcome the opportunity to engineer the perfection and implementation of a functional, comprehensive plan.

In healthcare facilities, nurse managers, occupational health nurses, laboratory managers, and other administrators must be prepared to accommodate all contingencies that can be reasonably anticipated. Those who work in capacities without immediate access to an occupational health nurse (e.g., physicians' offices, public health departments, home health agencies, etc.) must be aware of the decisions they will have to make in the event of an accidental exposure. Healthcare professionals can avoid the anxiety of making decisions while coping with the emotional trauma inherent in an exposure by preparing in advance and under calm circumstances. Preparedness can be assessed in a "trial run" in which an exposure is simulated, followed by the implementation of the postexposure protocol. By investing in anticipatory training when calm, rational thinking is possible, phlebotomists and other healthcare personnel with blood collection responsibilities can avoid the poor judgment and irrational decisions that can occur under the emotional trauma inherent in most exposures. This strategy also serves to reveal lapses in a facility's exposure control plan and gives managers an opportunity to improve the established protocol before a victim of an accidental needlestick is further victimized by postexposure chaos.

Some additional resources of interest include:

- Needlestick!
  http://www.needlestick.mednet.ucla.edu
- National Institute for Occupational Safety and Health, Centers for Disease Control and Prevention—bloodborne pathogens website
  http://www.cdc.gov/niosh/topics/bbp/
- Occupational Safety and Health Administration—bloodborne pathogens website
  http://www.osha-slc.gov/SLTC/bloodbornepathogens/indes.html
- National Clinicians' Postexposure Prophylaxis Hotline (PEPline)
  Phone: 888-448-4911 (24 hours/7 days a week)
  http://www.ucsf.edu/hivcntr/PEPline/
- Association for Professionals in Infection Control and Epidemiology, Inc.
  http://www.apic.org
- APIC Text of Infection Control and Epidemiology, R Carrico, ed. 2nd Revised Edition, Washington DC, 2005.

REFERENCES

1. Centers for Disease Control and Prevention Website. http://www.cdc.gov/sharpssafety/workbook. html. Accessed February 4, 2005.
2. Centers for Disease Control and Prevention. Updated U.S. Public Health Service guidelines for the management of occupational exposures to HBV, HCV, and HIV and recommendations for postexposure prophylaxis. *MMWR Morb Mortal Wkly Rep* 1 2001; 50(RR-11):1–52.
3. US Department of Labor, Occupational Health and Safety Administration. Occupational exposure to bloodborne pathogens; final rule. CFR part 1910.1030. *Federal Register* 1991; 56:64004–64182.
4. Godin G, Naccache H, Morel S, et al. Determinants of nurses' adherence to universal precautions for venipunctures. *Am J Infect Control* 2000;28:359–364.
5. Centers for Disease Control. Recommendations for prevention of HIV transmission in health-care settings. *MMWR Morb Mortal Wkly Rep* 1 1994;43(RR-11).
6. Centers for Disease Control. Update: universal precautions for prevention of transmission of human immunodeficiency virus, hepatitis B virus, and other bloodborne pathogens in health-care settings. *MMWR Morb Mortal Wkly Rep* 1 1988;37:377–382; 387–8.
7. Centers for Disease Control and Prevention. Immunization of healthcare workers: recommendations of the Advisory Committee on Immunization Practices (AICP) and the Hospital Infection Control Practices Advisory Committee (HICPAC). *MMWR Morb Mortal Wkly Rep* 1997;46(RR-18):1–42.
8. DeCock KM, Janssen RS. An unequal epidemic in an unequal world. *JAMA* 2002;228: 236.
9. Holding R. Carlsen W. Watchdogs fail health workers. *San Francisco Chronicle* 1998 April 12. Available at: http://www.sfgate.com (accessed June 8, 1998).
10. International Healthcare Worker Safety Center. Risk of infection following a single HIV, HBV, or HCV-contaminated needlestick or sharp instrument injury. Available at http://www.healthsystem.virginia.edu/internet/epinet/epinet4.cfm (accessed February 4, 2005).
11. Vidmar O, Poljak M, Tomazic J, et al. Transmission of HIV-1 by human bite [Letter]. *Lancet* 1996;347:1762–1763.

12. Lok AS, McMahon BJ. Chronic hepatitis B. *Hepatology* 2001;34:1225–1241.
13. Centers for Disease Control and Prevention. Protection against viral hepatitis: recommendations of the Advisory Committee on Immunization Practices (ACIP). *MMWR Morb Mortal Wkly Rep* 1990;39(RR-2):1–27.
14. Puro V, Petrosillo N, Ippolito G, Italian Study Group on Occupational Risk of HIV and Other Bloodborne Infections. Risk of hepatitis C seroconversion after occupational exposure in health care workers. *Am J Infect Control* 1995;23:273–277.
15. Beltrami EM, Kozak A, Williams IT, et al. Transmission of HIV and hepatitis C virus from a nursing home patient to a health care worker. *Am J Infect Control* 2003; 31:168–175.
16. National Institutes of Health Consensus Development Conference Panel Statement: Management of Hepatitis C. *Hepatology* 2002;36:S3–S20.
17. Centers for Disease Control and Prevention. Surveillance of healthcare personnel with HIV/AIDS, as of December 2001. Fact sheet. Available at: http://www.cdc.gov/ncidod/hip/Blood/hivpersonnel.htm. Accessed June 1, 2004.

Practices and Products for Exposure Prevention

9

INTRODUCTION

Hundreds of thousands of accidental needlesticks occur every year in the United States (Fig. 9.1). According to a United States General Accounting Office (GAO) projection, legislation mandating the use of safety needles in 2001 is expected to prevent at least 69,000 accidental needlesticks each year. Studies show that the accidental needlestick rates are declining as predicted, yet millions of healthcare workers remain at risk of acquiring any of the 20 different diseases reported to be transmitted by blood exposure because of unsafe practices (1–3).

As more healthcare workers assume phlebotomy responsibilities, it is becoming increasingly important to realize that protective products alone will not reduce accidental needlestick rates to their lowest possible level. Only through a combination of safe products *and practices* will a facility realize its greatest reduction in accidental exposures. Proper training in the use of safety devices must include those high-risk behaviors that increase the likelihood of sustaining an accidental needlestick. Those responsible for implementing and enforcing a facility's exposure control plan are obligated to regularly monitor the staff's adherence to safety policies and discipline those who engage in risky practices.

The risk is not limited to those who perform specimen collection procedures. For those who process and transport specimens, other means of exposure include:

- Tube breakage during centrifugation
- Tube breakage during transportation
- Splashes and spills when caps are removed
- Spills or splashes while transferring serum or plasma to a transport tube
- Splashes to the eye or nonintact skin during spill cleanup

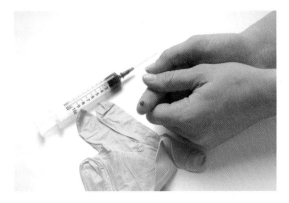

FIGURE 9.1 Hundreds of thousands of accidental needlesticks occur every year in the U.S.

This chapter discusses safe practices and how lax enforcement can contribute to preventable disease transmission. Also included is a rundown of products currently available that address needlestick safety.

After reading this chapter, the reader should be able to:

■ Discuss standard precautions
■ List practices that increase one's risk of exposure
■ Discuss the proper means of disposing contaminated sharps
■ Describe the appropriate use of personal protective equipment (PPE)
■ List products currently available designed to protect against accidental needlesticks

SAFE PRACTICES

Although sharps with safety features are widely used, safe products alone are not sufficient to fully protect healthcare workers from accidental exposures. Those who recap needles, dismantle safety features, draw blood without gloves, or perform other dangerous practices must be identified, disciplined, and retrained in order for a facility to properly manage infection control and employee safety. As identified in the Occupational Health and Safety Administration's (OSHA) Bloodborne Pathogens Standard, a thorough understanding of universal precautions (now referred to as "standard precautions"), the use of PPE, cleanup of biohazardous spills, and the handling of contaminated needles is critical for all healthcare workers with blood collection and processing responsibilities. Safe centrifuge use is also important to prevent exposures to contaminated glass shards and aerosols.

Standard Precautions

Standard precautions is a method of infection control in which all human blood and certain body fluids are treated as if known to be infectious for bloodborne pathogens (see Chapter 3). One study shows that nurses have a high intention of using universal precautions, but only 16 % admitted to using universal precautions in each of the last ten venipunctures they performed (3). Standards and recommendations from the Centers for Disease Control and Prevention (CDC) and OSHA include practices reflecting standard precautions (4, 5):

- Wash hands before and after patient care or if bodily fluids have been handled. According to the Bloodborne Pathogens Standard, "Employers shall ensure that employees wash their hands immediately or as soon as feasible after removal of gloves or other personal protective equipment." The CDC makes a similar recommendation in their revised guideline for hand hygiene (6). Because gloves are required for phlebotomy, these regulations mean hands must be washed between patients. If handwashing facilities are not available or if hands are not visibly soiled, alcohol-based hand-rubs and gels are acceptable substitutes (6). These guidelines have not only been established for the protection of the healthcare worker, but to prevent the spread of pathogens from patient to patient.
- Place intact needles, syringe units, and/or sharps in a designated disposal container as soon as possible without recapping. Studies show that 62 % of all accidental needlesticks occur within moments of when the needle is removed from the patient (7). OSHA mandates that safety features be activated immediately and the collection assembly be immediately discarded as one unit. (Fig. 9.2). Removing the needle is in violation of the Bloodborne Pathogens Standards and should not be performed unless the procedure requires it (e.g., removing a needle to attach a safety transfer device as in blood culture collection or when performing blood gas analysis) (see Box 9.1).
- Do not break or bend needles. Devices that bend or break needles are forbidden by OSHA regulations. In its compliance directive to inspectors detailing how the Bloodborne Pathogens Standard should be enforced, OSHA instructs, "Shearing or breaking of contaminated sharps is completely prohibited. . . (8)." Such manipulation subjects the collector to risk of exposure and generates aerosols that can be potentially infectious.

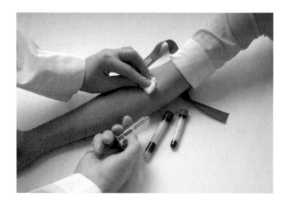

FIGURE 9.2 OSHA mandates that safety features be immediately activated and the assembled device be immediately discarded.

BOX 9.1   OSHA and Tube Holder Reuse

In 1991, the Bloodborne Pathogens Standard stated that "contaminated needles and other contaminated sharps shall not be bent, recapped, or removed," but lack of enforcement and vaguely worded exceptions allowed the practice of removing needles from tube holders and the subsequent reuse of the holder to continue unabated. In 2001, the agency issued a compliance directive on the Bloodborne Pathogens Standard (instructions to their inspectors on how to enforce various standards) establishing their position on removing needles from tube holders, "Devices with needles must be used and immediately discarded. . . (8)."

In 2002, OSHA issued a *Letter of Clarification* prohibiting tube holder reuse outright. The letter and its companion, *Letter of Interpretation,* removed any doubt regarding the agency's stance on removing needles from tube holders. "We want to make it clear that the practice is prohibited," says John Henshaw, OSHA's Administrator (9). According to the Letter of Interpretation, "In order to prevent potential worker exposure to the contaminated hollow-bore needle at both the front and back ends, blood tube holders, with needles attached, must be immediately discarded into an accessible sharps container after the safety feature has been activated (9)."

In 2003, OSHA issued a Safety and Health Information Bulletin (SHIB) reiterating their stance, "OSHA has concluded that the best practice for prevention of needlestick injuries following phlebotomy procedures is the use of a sharp with engineered sharps injury protection (SESIP) (e.g., safety needle) attached to the blood tube holder and the immediate disposal of the entire unit after each patient's blood is drawn (10)." According to Henshaw, "Single-use blood tube holders, when used with engineering and work practice controls, simply provide the best level of protection against needlestick injures. That is why the standard generally prohibits removing needles and reusing blood tube holders."

In the bulletin, OSHA recognizes that hazardous work practices continue to injure workers even though engineering controls—like needles with sharps injury protection features—are widely used. "The manipulation required to remove a contaminated needle, even a safety-engineered needle, from a blood tube holder may result in a needlestick with the back end of the needle, which is only covered with a rubber sleeve (10)."

■ Refrain from all direct patient care and handling patient care equipment if you have a weeping rash. Direct transmission of infectious agents to and from weeping rashes doubles the risk of spreading disease. Healthcare workers put themselves at risk of acquiring infections from patient surfaces while putting patients at risk of acquiring the organism causing the weeping rash.

Use of Personal Protective Equipment

Personal protective equipment (PPE), such as gloves, gowns, facemasks, and eye protection, is required when observing standard precautions. These devices protect both patient and healthcare worker from exposure and potential infection. OSHA establishes the necessity of PPE in the Bloodborne Pathogens Standard. The following are some of the agency's required use of PPEs during specimen collection and processing:

- Wearing gloves whenever contact with body substances, mucous membranes, or nonintact skin is possible (Fig. 9.3). This includes phlebotomy. According to OSHA, "Gloves shall be worn . . . when performing vascular access procedures. . . (5)." The only exception provided is for phlebotomists in a volunteer blood donation center (trainees are not exempt). OSHA's instructions to inspectors state, "At a minimum, gloves must be used . . . when performing vascular access procedures (8)." Glove use is also required whenever it can be reasonably expected that the healthcare worker could be exposed to blood or other potentially infectious materials, for example, when removing the caps from tubes during processing or when handling tubes and other specimen containers that are visibly contaminated.

Gloves cannot provide protection without decreasing sensitivity and, therefore, the ability to palpate the vein, but it is a necessary compromise. Healthcare personnel should become accustomed to the use of gloves and employ techniques that maintain glove use while minimizing their limitations. This can be accomplished by locating the vein prior to putting on the gloves. According to the Clinical and Laboratory Standards Institute, gloves need not be put on until after the vein has been located (with the exception of patients in isolation). To eliminate the need to repalpate the cleansed site after the gloves have been put on, make a mental note during the initial survey as to where the vein lies in relation to certain skin markers such as freckles, skin creases, or other surface features. After the gloves have been put on, these landmarks make relocation by palpation less necessary.

The frequent practice of tearing off the tip of the glove to expose the index finger circumvents the collector's safety and is in violation of OSHA's Bloodborne Pathogen Standard. Such practices subject the employer to fines and citations and should invoke disciplinary measures. (See Fig. 7.1, Chapter 7.)

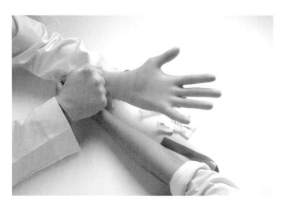

FIGURE 9.3 OSHA mandates that gloves be worn when performing vascular access procedures including phlebotomy.

Repeated use of latex gloves can lead to latex sensitivity in 6% to 17% of latex glove users (11). As a result, most facilities have moved, or are in transition, from latex to vinyl, nitrile, or other nonlatex gloves.

■ Wearing gowns impermeable to liquids when clothing is likely to become soiled or contaminated with body fluids. OSHA states that impermeable gowns must be worn when an exposure can be reasonably anticipated. Those who draw blood specimens must evaluate the potential for blood or other potentially infectious material to come in contact with their clothing with each patient and wear the appropriate protection. It has been reported that blood sprays from fingersticks and venipunctures can contaminate the collector from the tips of the fingers to the elbows and from the collarbone to the waist (12). OSHA consultants recommend lab coats with knitted cuffs for staff performing phlebotomies, with the gloves pulled over the cuffs to cover exposed skin.

It is also reasonable to anticipate this potential when the processing of blood specimens involves removing the stopper. The same potential exists when handling specimens visibly contaminated with blood (e.g., body fluids). Processing specimens without protective lab coats subjects the employee to the potential for contaminating the clothing they wear home to their families. Because hepatitis B can live on contaminated surfaces for up to 1 week, healthcare personnel put their families at risk of exposure when choosing not to wear impermeable lab coats while handling specimens (13).

According to OSHA, it is the responsibility of the employer to provide and launder impermeable gowns and to replace those in which the integrity of the barrier is compromised.

 Tips from the Trenches: *Because hepatitis B can live on contaminated surfaces for up to 1 week, healthcare workers put their families at risk of exposure when choosing not to wear impermeable lab coats while handling specimens.*

■ Wearing a mask and protective eyewear or a face shield when the risk of being splashed with body fluids exists. Those who collect and process blood specimens must evaluate the potential for eye splashes and use the proper equipment. Generally, specimen collection is not associated with the risk of eye exposure, but in those circumstances in which it can be reasonably anticipated, protection must be used in the form of eyewear or a protective shield positioned between the specimen and the face.

Specimen-processing personnel who remove stoppers from blood specimens should use protective equipment when exposure can be reasonably anticipated. Eyewear or a barrier between the specimen and the processor, such as a clear acrylic shield, can be used to prevent exposure due to the splattering of blood when specimens are uncapped and handled.

Proper Protocol for Accidental Blood Spills

Although use of plastic blood collection tubes is becoming more widespread, blood collection personnel may still be at risk for exposures due to broken glass. To minimize the risk, blood spills should be cleaned up immediately with gloves and other necessary PPE in place (Fig. 9.4). For small spills and splashes that do not involve broken glass, the area should be flooded with a solution of 10% bleach and wiped with absorbent towels (14). The towels should be discarded into a receptacle for biohazardous waste.

For large spills and/or spills involving broken glass, the spill should be flooded with 10% bleach and sprinkled with an absorbent compound. Commercial spill kits are available that contain gloves, a scoop, disinfectant wipes, a biohazardous waste bag, and an absorbent powder that congeals spills (EZ-Cleans Plus, SafeTec, Buffalo, NY, USA). To remove the hazard, sweep the broken glass and blood-soaked absorbent compound into a dustpan and discard into a sharps container. Flood the surface again with the bleach solution and wipe with absorbent towels. Discard towels into a biohazardous receptacle.

If a specimen tube breaks during centrifugation, keep the lid closed for at least 30 minutes to allow aerosols and fine droplets to settle. Then open the centrifuge carefully while wearing appropriate PPE and remove the larger pieces of glass with a hemostat or other device. Hands, even if gloved, should never be used to retrieve broken glass. Inspect other tubes in the centrifuge for damage and contamination. If the exterior of other tubes have been visibly contaminated, cleanse them with a solution of 10% bleach. Likewise, decontaminate the interior of the centrifuge (15). The use of puncture-resistant gloves is recommended.

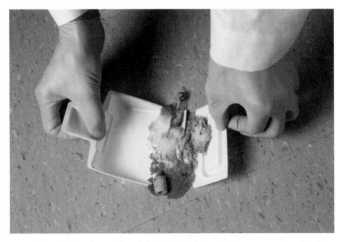

FIGURE 9.4 Broken glass contaminated with blood should be immediately cleaned up with the necessary personal protective equipment in place.

Proper Handling of Contaminated Needles

Conventional hollow-bore needles account for 68% of all accidental needle-sticks to healthcare workers (16). The CDC has shown that the use of safety needles and collection devices can reduce the frequency of accidental needle-sticks by up to 76% (7). Although the use of safer sharps is widespread, improper handling of sharps can still subject healthcare workers to unnecessary risk. (See "Respect the Needle," in the Phlebotomy Tip of the Month section, Appendix IV.)

As soon as the needle is removed from the patient, the healthcare worker is vulnerable to an accidental needlestick and remains vulnerable until the sharp is discarded. If the needle is not immediately discarded, concealed, destroyed, or otherwise rendered incapable of causing a puncture, the potential to acquire a life-threatening illness increases dramatically. Without exception, activating the device's safety feature must be instantaneous as the sharp is removed from the patient. Some devices even activate before being removed from the vein. (See "Safety Products," this chapter.)

After the blood has been obtained, remove the needle from the patient, activate the safety feature, and discard the device without disassembly in one fluid motion. An exception is if collecting blood by syringe (Fig. 9.5). Under this circumstance, the safety feature should be activated immediately, the needle removed, discarded, and replaced with a safety transfer device to fill the tubes.

Needle recapping must not be performed. Although OSHA allows recapping "when no alternative is feasible," managers must justify the practice in their facility's exposure control manual and support the practice with "reliable evidence (8)." The basis for the justification must then meet the inspector's satisfaction.

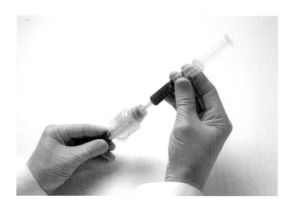

FIGURE 9.5 Safety transfer devices should be used when transferring blood from a syringe to specimen collection tubes

Safe Centrifuge Use

Blood specimen collection tubes should be capped during centrifugation to prevent aerosols from being emitted. Centrifuges should have a locking lid to prevent splatter and aerosols from escaping in the event a tube breaks during centrifugation. The locking mechanism should prevent opening of the lid while the rotor is in motion. For optimum protection, safety features on the centrifuge must be in place and activated. Modification or dismantling of safety features puts the healthcare professional at risk and is in violation of OSHA regulations.

SAFETY PRODUCTS

Because of the high rate of accidental needlesticks sustained by healthcare workers, the Needlestick Safety and Prevention Act was signed into law in 2000 instructing OSHA to revise the Bloodborne Pathogens Standard to require the use of sharps with engineered sharps injury protection (SESIP) features. Since 1988, the US Patent and Trademark Office has issued more

Unsafe Practices

Healthcare professionals must always guard against the temptation to use unsafe practices. The responsibility to prevent accidental exposure rests not only with the individual, but also with co-workers and managers. Those who observe violations to the Bloodborne Pathogens Standard are morally obligated to report infractions; those with supervisory responsibilities are likewise obligated to discipline employees who put themselves and their employer at risk by violating OSHA regulations and facility protocol. When managers and co-workers fail to address unsafe practices, they share in the responsibility should the employee eventually be exposed or acquire a bloodborne disease. The following practices should be reported and lead to disciplinary action:

- Drawing blood without gloves or with gloves of compromised integrity (e.g., with the tips of the fingers cut off)
- Recapping a needle
- Using a conventional, nonsafety needle
- Dismantling or removing safety features from needles and other blood collection devices
- Failure to immediately activate the safety feature of a needle
- Allowing a sharps container to fill beyond capacity
- Not wearing an impermeable gown or providing for eye protection when removing stoppers from collection tubes
- Not using a safety transfer device when transferring blood from a syringe to collection tubes
- Use of nonretractable skin puncture lancets
- Cleaning any blood spill without gloves and major spills without gloves and impermeable gowns
- Failure to report infractions

than 1,000 patents for devices that protect healthcare workers from accidental needlesticks (17). As a result, a multitude of new products continue to emerge to minimize the healthcare professional's exposure to contaminated sharps. OSHA mandates that those in a position to evaluate and implement safety products consider new products annually and document such consideration in their exposure control plan (5).

The list of products that address exposure prevention is extensive. Although it is beyond the scope of this text to list them all, what follows is a market survey of many of the most commonly used devices and products designed to reduce healthcare worker exposure to bloodborne pathogens. Categories include:

- Sharps with engineered SESIPs
- Needle disposal units
- Needle destruction units
- Laser skin perforation devices

Engineered Sharps Injury Protection

In the revised Bloodborne Pathogens Standard, OSHA requires "engineering controls" be implemented to reduce employee exposure. OSHA defines engineering controls as "controls (e.g., sharps disposal containers, self-sheathing needles, safer medical devices, such as sharps with engineered sharps injury protections and needleless systems) that isolate or remove the bloodborne pathogens hazard from the workplace." Sharps with SESIPs are further defined as "a nonneedle sharp or a needle device used for withdrawing body fluids, accessing a vein or artery, or administering medications or other fluids, with a built-in safety feature or mechanism that effectively reduces the risk of an exposure incident."

This section discusses the various SESIPs available to comply with OSHA regulations at the time of publication. Manufacturers of specimen collection supplies and equipment continue to develop products and improve on existing technologies with a priority given to the desirable characteristics of safety devices as recommended by the National Institute of Occupational Safety and Health (NIOSH) (18). Those characteristics include:

- The device is needleless
- The safety feature is an integral part of the device
- The device preferably works passively (i.e., it requires no activation by the user). If user activation is necessary, the safety feature can be engaged with a single-handed technique and allows the worker's hands to remain behind the exposed sharp
- The user can easily tell whether the safety feature is activated
- The safety feature cannot be deactivated and remains protective through disposal
- The device performs reliably
- The device is easy to use and practical
- The device is safe and effective for patient care

The NIOSH recommendation for single-handed activation is critical to safety. An activation feature used while the needle is still in the vein and/or requires one hand to activate provides the greatest safety and convenience. With one hand applying pressure on the puncture site, any device requiring two hands to activate incorporates a dangerous delay in the process and is inherently disadvantageous.

Although not a comprehensive list of safety products on the market, Table 9.1 presents some of the current designs available to protect the healthcare professional from the risks involved in blood specimen collection.

Needle Disposal Units

A needle disposal unit (sharps container) must be on the tray of blood collection supplies or positioned within reach (5). Units positioned away from the patient and that require the collector to carry a contaminated sharp any distance from the point of use are ineffective and put the healthcare worker at great risk. According to the Bloodborne Pathogens Standard, "contaminated sharps shall be discarded immediately or as soon as feasible in containers that are closable, puncture resistant, leak proof on sides and bottom and labeled or color-coded" in accordance with OSHA labeling standards (5). They should remain upright throughout use and not be allowed to overfill.

In 2003, OSHA issued a Safety and Health Information Bulletin (SHIB) discussing the agency's stance on making sharps containers available at the point of use (10). The bulletin states "employees must have access to sharps containers that are easily accessible to the immediate area where sharps are used" (Fig. 9.6). A warning issued in the bulletin recognizes that not all sharps containers allow disposal of a sharp attached to the collection device. These containers are not in compliance with the Bloodborne Pathogens Standard, "Employers must ensure that where blood is being drawn, the sharps container is appropriate for immediate disposal of sharps."

It Could Happen to You

A healthcare professional, just beginning his shift, found the sharps container on the phlebotomy tray filled to capacity. Closing the unit required him to press a hinged flap over the top opening and lock it into place. The container was so full that closing the flaps required squeezing the lid with significant force, using both hands. The pressure necessary to lock the lid forced a contaminated sharp through the bottom of the container, piercing his thumb.

Question: How could this injury have been prevented?

Answer: When needle disposal units are three-fourths full, they should be sealed and discarded according to the facility's protocol for disposal. Units that are allowed to fill beyond this level put healthcare professionals at risk for accidental needlesticks.

TABLE 9.1 Safety Products

Modified Tube Holders

VanishPoint	Retractable Technologies	(888) 703-1010	www.vanish-point.com
Venipuncture Needle-Pro	Sims Portex	(800) 258-5361	www.portexusa.com
Saf-T Holder	Sims Portex	(800) 258-5361	www.portexusa.com
Saf-T Closed Blood Collection System™	Sims Portex	(800) 258-5361	www.portexusa.com
ProGuard II	Kendall	(508) 261-8027	www.kendallhq.com
Defender	Kendall	(508) 261-8027	www.kendallhq.com
QuickShield	Greiner Bio-One	(888) 286-3883	www.vacuette.com

Modified Needles

Punctur-Gard	ICU Medical	(800) 824-7890	www.icumed.com
Monoject Magellan	Monoject, a division of Kendall	(508) 261-8027	www.kendallhq.com
SurGuard2	Terumo	(800) 283-7866	www.terumomedical.com
Eclipse	BD	(800) 595-0257	www.bd.com
Safe-Point Vac	North American Medical Products (NAMP)	(800) 488-6267	(no web site)

Winged Blood Collection Sets

Safety Blood Collection Sets	Greiner Bio-One	(888) 286-3883	www.vacuette.com
Angel Wing	Kendall	(508) 261-8027	www.kendallhq.com
Wingset	ICU Medical	(800) 824-7890	www.icumed.com
Safety-Lok	BD	(800) 595-0257	www.bd.com
Vaku-8 Plus	Myco Medical	(919) 678-0680	
Surshield Safety Winged Blood Collection Set	Terumo	(800) 283-7866	www.terumomedical.com
Saf-T Wing Infusion Set	Sims Portex	(800) 258-5361	www.portexusa.com
Push Button Blood Collection Set	BD	(800) 595-0257	www.bd.com

Other Blood Collection Systems

S-Monovette	Sarstedt	(800) 257-5101	sarstedt.com

Needle Destruction Units (NDU)

Needlyzer	MedPro	(859) 225-5375	www.needlyzer.com
SharpX	Bio Medical Disposal	(888) 393-9595	www.biodisposal.com

Laser Skin Perforation Devices

Lasette	Cell Robotics International	(505) 343-1131	www.cellrobotics.com
Laser Lancet	Transmedica		www.transmedicainc.com

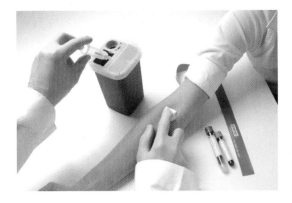

FIGURE 9.6 Tube holders with needles must be discarded at the point of use without disassembly.

Needle Destruction Units

Needle Destruction Units (NDU) allow one-handed needle disposal by disintegrating the needle immediately after use in a process known as pyroelectric oxidation. When removed from the vein, the contaminated needle is immediately inserted into the NDU, which activates the device, reducing the sharp to a metallic ash that falls into a catch bin. Such devices allow for one-handed needle disposal at the point of use, significantly reducing the volume of waste in sharps containers. NDUs are recognized by OSHA as sharps disposal units, not SESIPs. In hospital settings, these devices are contraindicated in areas where potentially explosive gases (oxygen, etc.) or liquids are being used or stored.

Laser Skin Perforation Devices

For patients who perform home glucose monitoring as well as healthcare professionals who perform skin puncture procedures, laser skin perforation devices are available for needleless punctures that minimize the discomfort and the risk of exposure. Laser perforation devices vaporize up to 2 mm of the skin with a tightly focused pulse of light energy, yielding blood in quantities sufficient for most bedside testing. Patients feel a sensation of mild heat or pressure instead of the sharp pain of a traditional puncturing device. Such devices eliminate the risk of accidental needlesticks during capillary punctures because they negate the use of lancets when small quantities of blood are required. Wounds have been reported to heal faster than those inflicted by lancets when produced by these devices (16). Laser skin perforation devices are not recommended in areas where oxygen is in use.

Needlestick Injury Statistics

The following statistics underscore the importance of protecting the healthcare professional against accidental exposure:

- Needlesticks by occupation (18,19)
  Nurses: 46%
  Laboratory technicians: 23%
  Doctors: 15%
  Housekeeper/laundry: 5%
  Other: 12%
- Chance of becoming infected when stuck with a contaminated needle (16,20)
  Hepatitis B: 30%
  Hepatitis C: 1.8%
  HIV: 1 in 300
- Estimated accidental needlestick injuries sustained by healthcare workers worldwide per year: 1 million (16,20)
- Number of accidental needlesticks that go unreported: up to 92% (20)
- Accidental needlesticks per day: 2,400
- Percent of accidental needlesticks caused by hollow-bore needles: 68% (16)
- Healthcare workers projected to be infected with HIV through accidental needlesticks per year: 18 to 60 (21)
- Healthcare personnel infected with hepatitis B every year from accidental needlesticks: 1,000 (21)
- Number of diseases capable of being transmitted through needlesticks: at least 20 (2)
- Cost of treating accidental needlestick (testing and prophylaxis): $4,000 (16)
- Cost of treating HIV-infected employee (from needlestick): $500,000 to $1 million (22)
- Average legal settlement for occupationally acquired HIV: $2 to $5 million (20)

REFERENCES

1. Study shows needlestick injuries on the gradual decline. *Inf Ctl Today* 2003;7:39–42.
2. Jagger J. Rates of needlestick injury caused by various devices in a university hospital. *N Engl J Med* 1988;319:284–288.
3. Godin G, Naccache H, Morel S, et al. Determinants of nurses' adherence to standard precautions for venipunctures. *AJIC* 2000;28:359–364.
4. Ernst D, Ernst C. *Phlebotomy for nurses and nursing personnel.* Ramsey, IN: HealthStar Press, 2001.
5. US Department of Labor and Occupational Safety and Health Administration (OSHA). Occupational exposure to bloodborne pathogens: final rule (29 CFR 1910.1030). *Federal Register* 1991;Dec 6:64004–64182.
6. Centers for Disease Control and Epidemiology. Guideline for hand hygiene in healthcare settings. *MMWR Morb Mortal Wkly Rep* 2002;51(RR16):1–44.
7. Centers for Disease Control and Prevention. Evaluation of safety devices for preventing percutaneous injuries among health-care workers during phlebotomy procedures. *MMWR Morb Mortal Wkly Rep* 1997;46:21–25.

8. US Department of Labor and Occupational Safety and Health Administration (OSHA). Enforcement Procedures for Occupational Exposure to Bloodborne Pathogens. CPL 2-2.69. http://www.osha-slc.gov/pls/oshaweb/owadisp.show_document?p_table=DIRECTIVES&p_id=2570 (accessed 2/22/04).

9. Occupational Safety and Health Administration. *Standard interpretation: reuse of tube holders.* http://www.osha.gov/pls/oshaweb/owadisp.show_document?p_table=INTERPRETATIONS&p_id=24040 (accessed 7/1/04).

10. Occupational Safety and Health Administration. *Safety Health and Information Bulletin.*

11. ECRI. Latex Sensitivity: Clinical and Legal Issues. *The Risk Management Reporter* August 1997.

12. Lusky K. Rooting out 'invisible' blood collection errors. *CAP Today* 2003;17:26–31.

13. Center for Disease Control updates public health guidelines for managing exposure to HBV, HCV and HIV. *Lab Med* 2001;32:495–501.

14. NCCLS. *Protection of laboratory workers from occupationally acquired infections; approved guideline—second edition.* NCCLS document M29-A2. Wayne, PA, 2001.

15. NCCLS. *Protection of laboratory workers from instrument biohazards and infectious disease transmitted by blood, body fluids, and tissue.* Approved Guideline M29-A. Villanova, PA, 1997.

16. Carlsen W, Holding R. Epidemic ravages caregivers; Thousands die from diseases contracted through needle sticks. *San Francisco Chronicle* 1998, April 12.

17. Carlsen W, Holding R. Safety designs proposed but not produced. *San Francisco Chronicle* 1998, April 12.

18. CDC. *NIOSH alert: preventing needlestick injuries in health care settings.* DHS Publication no. 2000-108 (NIOSH). Cincinnati, OH: Department of Health and Human Services, CDC, 1999. http://www.osha.gov/pls/oshaweb/owadisp.show_document?p_table=NEWS_RELEASES&p_id=10495 (accessed 3/11/04).

19. Kearsly S. High profits—at what cost? *San Francisco Chronicle* 1998, April 14.

20. Pallatroni L. Needlesticks: who pays the price when costs are cut on safety? *MLO* 1998; 30:30.

21. Holding R, Carlsen W. Watchdogs fail health workers. *San Francisco Chronicle* 1998 April 12. Available at http://www.sfgate.com (accessed 6/8/98).

22. Statement by Secretary of Labor Alexis M. Herman on preventing needlestick injuries, May 20, 1999. Available at http://osha.gov/media/statements/ndlstmt052099.html (accessed May 21, 1999).

REVIEW QUESTIONS

1. In June of 2002, OSHA defined the intent of the Bloodborne Pathogens Standard as it applies to needle removal and subsequent tube holder reuse in a:
   a. Letter of Clarification
   b. Letter of Interpretation
   c. a and b
   d. compliance directive

2. In OSHA's recent Letter of Interpretation, "blood tube holders, with needles attached, must be immediately discarded into an accessible sharps container. . .:
   a. unless it can be demonstrated that the sharp is permanently shielded."
   b. after the safety feature has been activated."
   c. unless it is documented in the facility's exposure control plan that no alternative is feasible."
   d. or otherwise rendered incapable of causing an exposure."

3. According to a United States General Accounting Office (GAO) projection, legislation mandating the use of safety needles in 2001 should prevent at least _____ accidental needlesticks each year.
   a. 560,000
   b. 800,000
   c. 1 million
   d. 69,000

4. For healthcare facilities, achieving the greatest reduction in accidental exposures requires a combination of
   a. modified needles and modified tube holders
   b. SESIPs and sharps containers at the point of use
   c. safe products and safe practices
   d. safe products and regular monitoring of safety feature activation

5. According to OSHA's most recent clarification of the needle removal/tube holder reuse issue:
   a. tube holders can only be reused if there is no visible contamination
   b. tube holders with needles attached must be discarded without disassembly immediately after use
   c. tube holders can be washed in bleach and reused
   d. tube holders with automatic needle release mechanisms are exempt from the disposal requirement

6. Standard precautions is a method of infection control in which all human blood and certain body fluids are treated as if:
   a. known to be infectious for bloodborne pathogens
   b. they are sterile
   c. they have the potential to transmit hepatitis
   d. an OSHA inspector was observing

7. Studies show that 62% of all accidental needlesticks occur:
   a. within moments of when the needle is removed from the patient
   b. during nursing procedures

    c. to downstream waste handlers

    d. during activation of safety features

8. OSHA states that impermeable gowns must be worn:

    a. when drawing blood from patients

    b. when the blood being drawn or handled is known to be infected with bloodborne pathogens

    c. when drawing blood from combative patients

    d. when an exposure can be reasonably anticipated

9. According to OSHA, gloves shall be worn:

    a. whenever performing vascular access procedures unless not required by facility policy

    b. when processing specimens

    c. when performing vascular access procedures

    d. when drawing donor blood in volunteer blood donation facilities

10. Conventional hollow-bore needles account for 68% of all accidental needlesticks to

    a. healthcare workers

    b. nursing personnel

    c. physicians

    d. phlebotomists

11. Should a specimen tube break during centrifugation:

    a. quarantine the area until a hazardous materials cleanup crew removes the hazard

    b. remove the contaminated glass and clean the centrifuge immediately

    c. report the incident to the appropriate infection control personnel

    d. keep the lid closed for at least a half-hour to allow the aerosols and fine droplets to settle

12. One of the characteristics of safety devices recommended by the National Institute of Occupational Safety and Health (NIOSH) is that:

    a. the safety feature is an integral part of the device

    b. the sharp is retractable

    c. the device meets CDC standards

    d. the device is OSHA compliant

Clinical and Laboratory Standards Institute (formerly NCCLS) Documents

CLSI940 West Valley Road, Suite 1400
Wayne, PA 19087
Phone: 610-688-0100
Fax: 610-688-0700
Web address: www.clsi.org
E-mail: Exoffice@clsi.org

C38-A *Control of Analytic Variation in Trace Element Analysis; Approved Guideline (1997).* This document provides guidelines for patient preparation, specimen collection, transport, and processing for the analysis of trace metals in a variety of biological matrices.

H1-A5 *Evacuated Tubes and Additives for Blood Specimen Collection—Fifth Edition; Approved Standard (2003).* This document provides requirements for blood collection tubes and additives.

H3-A5 *Procedures for the Collection of Diagnostic Blood Specimens by Venipuncture—Fifth Edition; Approved Standard (2003).* This document provides procedures for the collection of diagnostic specimens by venipuncture, including line draws, blood culture collection, and venipuncture in children. It also includes recommendations on the order of draw.

H4-A5 *Procedures and Devices for the Collection of Diagnostic Capillary Blood Specimens—Fifth Edition; Approved Standard (2004).* This standard provides detailed descriptions and explanations of proper collection techniques, as well as hazards to patients from inappropriate specimen collection by skin puncture procedures.

H11-A4 *Procedure for the Collection of Arterial Blood Specimens—Fourth Edition; Approved Standard (2004).* This standard describes principles of collecting, handling, and transporting arterial blood specimens. The document is aimed at reducing collection hazards and ensuring integrity of the arterial specimen.

H18-A3 *Procedures for the Handling and Processing of Blood Specimens; Approved Guideline—Third Edition (2004).* This guideline addresses multiple factors associated with handling and processing specimens, as well as factors that can introduce imprecision or systematic bias into results.

H21-A4 *Collection, Transport, and Processing of Blood Specimen for Testing Plasma-Based Coagulation Assays—Fourth Edition; Approved Guideline (2003).* This guideline contains procedures for collecting, transporting, and storing blood; processing blood specimens; storing plasma for coagulation testing.

M29-A2 *Protection of Laboratory Workers from Occupationally Acquired Infections—Second Edition; Approved Guideline (2001).* This document provides guidance on the risk of transmission of hepatitis viruses and human immunodeficiency viruses in any laboratory setting, specific precautions for preventing the laboratory transmission of bloodborne infection from laboratory instruments and materials, and recommendations for the management of bloodborne exposure.

T/DM6-A *Blood Alcohol Testing in the Clinical Laboratory; Approved Guideline (1997).* This document gives technical and administrative guidance on laboratory procedures related to blood alcohol testing.

Recommended Certification Organizations

American Certification Agency (ACA)
PO Box 58
Osceola, IN 46561
Phone: 574-277-4538
Fax: 574-277-4624
Web address: www.acacert.com

Requirements to take written and practical test: high school diploma and
1. One year of experience OR
2. Successful completion of an approved phlebotomy program that includes didactic and minimum 100 clinical hours with completion of a minimum of 100 successful venipunctures.

Continuing education required to remain certified? Yes, every 2 years.

American Medical Technologists (AMT)
710 Higgins Road
Parkridge, IL 60068-5765
Phone: 847-823-5169 or 800-275-1268
Fax: 847-823-0458
Web address: www.amt1.com

Requirements to take written exam: high school diploma or equivalent and:
1. Graduation from a phlebotomy course in a school or program accredited by the Accrediting Bureau of Health Education Schools (ABHES) plus completion of a minimum of 50 venipunctures and 25 finger/heelsticks, OR
2. Graduation from an acceptable program in an institution accredited by an agency recognized by the United States Department of Education or the Commission on the Recognition of Postsecondary Accreditation (COPRA) plus completion of at least 50 venipunctures and 25 finger/heelsticks, OR

3. Successful completion of an acceptable phlebotomy training program, which includes at least 120 hours of clinical practical and a minimum of 50 venipunctures and 25 finger/heelsticks, OR

4. Completion of at least 1,040 hours of acceptable work experience as a phlebotomy technician within the past 3 years; this is to include at least 50 venipunctures, 25 skin punctures, specimen processing, communication skills, and clerical duties.

Examination waived if applicant:

1. Has passed a phlebotomist examination for the purpose of state licensure, OR

2. Holds other phlebotomy certification obtained by examination and is determined by the Board to have met the AMT training and experience requirements.

Continuing education required to remain certified? Yes.

American Society for Clinical Pathology Board of Registry (ASCP-BOR)
2100 West Harrison Street
Chicago, IL 60612
Phone: 312-738-1336
Fax:(312) 738-1619
Web address: www.ascp.org

Requirements to take written examination: high school diploma (or equivalent) and:

1. Completion of a National Accreditation Agency for Clinical Laboratory Science (NAACLS)-approved phlebotomy program within the last 5 years, OR

2. Completion of an acceptable formal structured phlebotomy program, which includes 120 clinical hours with a minimum performance of 100 successful venipunctures, 25 successful capillary punctures, observation of 5 arterial punctures, orientation in a full-service laboratory, and 40 clock-hours of didactic training at a regionally-accredited college/university or laboratory within the last 5 years, OR

3. One year of full-time experience as a phlebotomy technician in an accredited laboratory within the last 5 years, which included venipunctures, capillary punctures, observation of arterial punctures, and orientation in a full-service laboratory, OR

4. Completion of an accredited allied health professional/occupational education with phlebotomy training including performance of a minimum of 100 successful venipunctures, 25 successful capillary punctures, observation of five arterial punctures, and orientation in a full-service laboratory.

Continuing education required to remain certified? Yes, every 3 years.

National Credentialing Agency (NCA)
PO Box 15945-289
Lenexa, KS 66285
Phone: 913-438-5110 ext. 647
Fax: 913 599-5340
Web address: www.nca-info.org

Requirements to take written exam: high school diploma and:
1. Successful completion of an approved phlebotomy program that includes a clinical component in phlebotomy, OR
2. One year of full-time work experience including phlebotomy.

Continuing education required to remain certified? Yes, every 3 years.

National Center for Competency Testing (NCCT)
7007 College Boulevard, Suite 705
Overland Park, KS 66211
Phone: 913-498-1000
Fax: 913-498-1243
Web address: www.ncctinc.com

Requirements to take written exam: high school diploma or equivalent and:
1. Successful completion of an approved phlebotomy program or documentation of at least 1 year of experience as a phlebotomist and
2. Signed NCCT documentation of performance minimums.

Continuing education required to remain certified? Yes, annually.

National Healthcareer Association (NHA)
134 Evergreen Place, 9th Floor
East Orange, NJ 07018
Phone: 800-499-9092
Fax: 973-678-7305
Web address: www.nhanow.com

Requirements to take written exam: high school diploma or equivalent and
1. Successful completion of an approved phlebotomy program, OR
2. One year of phlebotomy experience.

Requirement for waiver from exam: 2 years of phlebotomy experience and completion of a home-study packet.

Continuing education required to remain certified? Yes, every 2 years.

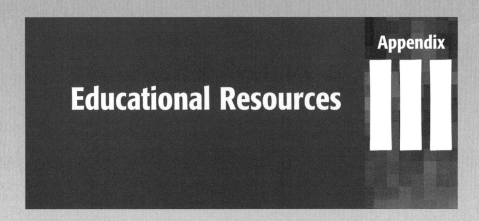

Educational Resources

Exam Review Guides
Phlebotomy Exam Review
Ruth E. McCall & Cathee Tankersley
Lippincott Williams & Wilkins
351 W. Camden Street.
Baltimore, MD 21201
Phone: 800-638-3030
Web address: www.lww.com

Question and Answer Review for Phlebotomy
Diana Garza & Kathleen Becan-McBride
Pearson Education
Upper Saddle River, NJ 07458
Web address: www.prenhall.com/healthprofessions

Organizations Offering Continuing Education in Phlebotomy
Center for Phlebotomy Education, Inc.
PO Box 161
Ramsey, IN 47166
Phone: 812-633-4636
Fax: 812-633-2346
Web address: www.phlebotomy.com
E-mail: phlebotomy@phlebotomy.com

American Society for Clinical Pathology
2100 West Harrison Street
Chicago, IL 60612
Phone: 312-738-1336
Fax:(312) 738-1619
Web address: www.ascp.org
E-mail: Info@ascp.org.

ABP, Inc.
PO Box 127
Granger, IN 46530
Phone: 800-500-0691
Fax: (574) 277-4624
Web address: www.abpincorp.com
E-mail: info@abpincorp.com

American Medical Technologists
710 Higgins Road
Park Ridge, IL 60068-5765
Phone: 800-275-1268
Fax: 847-823-0458
Web address: www.amt1.com
E-mail: mail@amt1.com

American Society for Clinical Laboratory Science
216710 Democracy Boulevard, Suite 300
Bethesda, MD 20817-1574
Phone: 301-657-2768
Fax: 301-657-2909
Web address: www.ascls.org
E-mail: elissap@ascls.org

Colorado Association for Continuing Medical Laboratory Education
6825 E. Tennessee Avenue, Suite 111
Denver, CO 80224
Phone: 303-321-1734
Fax: 303-321-9231
Web address: www.cacmle.org
E-mail: infor@cacmle.org

California Association for Medical Laboratory Technology
1895 Mowry Avenue, Suite 112
Fremont, CA 94538
Phone: 510-792-4441
Fax: 510-792-3045
Web address: www.camlt.org
E-mail: office@camlt.org

Clinical Laboratory Management Association
989 Old Eagle School Road, Suite 815
Wayne, PA 19087-1704
Phone: 610-995-9580
Fax: 610-995- 9568
Web address: www.clma.org
E-mail: wmetzgar@clma.org

HealthRx Corporation
7001B Loisdale Road, Springfield, VA 22150
Phone: 703-913-7900
Fax: 703-995-4632
Web address: www.etotallab.com
E-mail: etotallab@healthrx.com

National Center for Competency Testing (NCCT)
7007 College Boulevard
Overland Park, KS 66211
Phone: 913-498-1000
Fax: 913-498-1243
Web address: www.ncctinc.com

National Healthcareer Association (NHA)
134 Evergreen Place, 9th Floor
East Orange, NJ 07018
Phone: 800-499-9092
Fax: 973-678-7305
Web address: www.nhanow.com

University of Medicine and Dentistry of New Jersey
Center for Advanced and Continuing Education
1776 Raritan Road
Scotch Plains, NH 07748
Phone: 908-889-2560
Web address: ccoe.umdnj.edu/caceweb/overview.htm
E-mail: fydrysna@umdnj.edu

Appendix IV

Phlebotomy Tip of the Month

YOU ARE THE LAB!

What does it say about the skill of a tailor whose own suit doesn't fit? What does it say about the meal if the chef emerges from the kitchen picking his nose? Would you buy a diet book if you knew the author was 100 pounds overweight? Let's face it, we are walking advertisements for whatever it is we do. Like it or not, the image we project tells people something about us and the quality of work we produce. The old saying "you can't judge a book by its cover" is just flat-out wrong. Fair or not, you can and everyone does. So get used to being judged by your appearance and your personality.

If you draw blood for a laboratory, to the patient, you represent the lab. In the 5 minutes you spend with a patient, her impression of the quality of work conducted on her specimens is based completely and entirely on her impression of you. The way you dress, how you're groomed, your attitude, personality, and skill all combine to draw a picture of the laboratory. If the phlebotomist is sloppy, patients suspect that the laboratory is sloppy, too. If you are cold and inconsiderate, patients will suspect that the work performed on the specimen will be conducted carelessly. If the phlebotomist lacks skill, confidence, and professionalism, the patient will get the impression the rest of the laboratory is the same way. It's not fair, but that's the way it is. Get over it. You are the only source of information the patient gets on what the laboratory is like.

Is your lab coat or scrubs clean? Then so is the laboratory. Do you wear gloves when you draw blood? Then the laboratory must process the specimen carefully. Do you speak knowledgeably and considerately to the patient? Then the laboratory must be staffed with knowledgeable and considerate people.

Consider yourself to be the laboratory's ambassador. More than likely, your laboratory does exceptional work. Can your patients tell that by the way you look and interact with them? More than likely, your laboratory is staffed with highly skilled techs dedicated to producing accurate results in a timely fashion. Is that what patients sense when you leave their room? Patients never see the laboratory. As a phlebotomist, you wield significant power by being their representative. The patients' confidence that their specimen will be processed and tested properly depends on the 5 minutes or so that you spend with them.

WHAT IMAGE DO YOU PROJECT?

Dump the Baggage!

What is heavier than a phlebotomy tray, never appreciated by patients, makes our job miserable when we carry it around and is almost impossible to get rid of? Give up? Emotional baggage.

We all carry some around. Let's face it: life happens, and it isn't always pretty. Our significant others dump us; our teenagers defy us; our co-workers exploit us; our bosses pick on us; we're underpaid, underappreciated, under-loved, and overtaxed. The list of challenges to the human spirit is endless. The question is not if we'll have to suffer, it's when. And it's how. We can either work through those things that give us angst or we can be flat-out mis-erable to be around. When we choose to work through it, though, it can take weeks or months. But we will eventually get past it without dragging every-one down with us. But if we choose to seethe in anger, we tend to make oth-ers sorry they ever met us.

As healthcare professionals, we come in contact with strangers every day, most with a right to be more miserable than we are. It's not that dwelling on our problems isn't healthy. It's just that when we encounter patients, can't we just put it aside long enough to be nice? Regardless of how unfair life has been to you, the person on the other end of your needle needs you to be pleas-ant. Just for as long as it takes to draw blood, then you can go back to being miserable. Chances are your problems pale in comparison to those of your patients.

Make it a point that when you enter a patient's room, stop for a minute and leave your baggage at the door. Promise yourself that you will pick it up as soon as you are through being nice to the patient inside the room. Trust me; it'll be there waiting for you when you're done. Nobody else wants it. Do the same at the next door and the one after that until you can take it back with you from whence you came. Do this for a week. Then the next week, park your baggage at the entrance of the building where you work. Pick it up on your way out. It'll still be there for you to take home and share with your family. Then the week after that, enter work through a door that you've never used before. Park your baggage and never come back for it. You're bet-ter off without it. So are your patients, your friends, your family, and every stranger you'll ever meet. Really.

TREATING ALL PATIENTS AS IF THEY WERE FAMILY

When patients are admitted to hospitals or long-term care facilities, they are usually stripped of all of their belongings and much of their dignity. Personal valuables must be taken home or locked up for safekeeping; gowns are issued that seem designed to embarrass; strangers come and go without warning or a decent introduction wielding devices that poke, probe, and otherwise invade the body; privacy is not allowed; and permission often must be sought for activities that never needed permission at home, like using the rest room. It can be a discouraging and dehumanizing experience.

Healthcare workers are too often too overwhelmed by their own responsibilities to consider the impact hospitalization has on their patients. However, caregivers who weave a few basic courtesies into their approach can have a significant impact on their patients experience and, perhaps, the healing process. Treating all patients as if they are family is an attitude worth developing. To make your patients feel like they belong to your inner circle, try incorporating some of these considerations into your routine:

Introduce yourself—If you are not the patient's immediate caregiver, you are a stranger to the patient, and strangers should introduce themselves. Don't assume the patient doesn't care who you are or what you are up to. Telling patients your name and purpose also tells them that it is important to you that they feel comfortable with you.

Knock on the door—If you're new to the patient, knocking on the door says that you respect the few square feet that the patient has been assigned to as their turf. You don't have to wait for permission to enter, but a knock displays respect. It also serves as an announcement that can save the patient some embarrassment if he/she is in the middle of a "bodily function."

Leave your attitude behind—We all carry baggage. Emotions ebb and flow within us as life's dramas unfold in our own lives. Sometimes it's more than we can handle to keep it hidden within. However trivial or tragic, patients have their hands full dealing with their own problems without having to deal with ours at the same time. They don't care what we're going through; they just want us to perform our function skillfully without feeling like they are a burden. Smile.

Leave the room the way you found it—Bedridden patients depend on having their items within reach. If you've moved the bedside tray aside to perform a venipuncture, return it before you leave the room. Failure to do so can cause patients to fall should they try to retrieve it themselves.

Say "Thanks"—No explanation necessary.

ARE CALLERS GLAD YOU ANSWERED?

When you answer the phone, are callers glad you answered or do they wish someone else had? How about when you place a call? Take this simple test and find out how your phone manners rate.

1. When you answer the phone in your workplace, do you identify your-self and your department?
   Yes = 5 points   No = 0 points

   This is basic customer service and telephone etiquette. It's polite, it's professional, and it tells the caller they dialed the right number. When you sound professional on the other end of the line, people naturally form a higher opinion of you, your department, and the quality of work you both are capable of. Everyone knows that if you want to be considered a professional, you have to act like one. That includes how you answer the phone.

2. When you place a call, do you identify yourself, who you are with, and the nature of your call?
   Yes = 5 points   No = 0 points

   Even the most annoying creatures on earth, telemarketers, identify themselves when they call, and you're waaaay above them on the evolutionary ladder. Even if it's a department you call frequently, don't assume the person on the other end knows the sound of your voice.

3. When you place someone on hold, do you keep their wait at less than 1 minute?
   Yes = 5 points   No = 0 points

   Callers don't like to think they've been forgotten. If you think you'll have to keep a caller on hold longer than 1 minute, ask if you can call back when you have the information. Too much time spent waiting is a time killer that makes callers anxious at best, cranky at worst.

4. Do I answer each call within three rings?
   Yes = 5 points   No = 0 points

   This is kinda obvious, isn't it?

5. Do you end every call with "Thank-You. Goodbye?"
   Yes = 5 points   No = 0 points

   Abruptly ending a conversation without signing off is cold and tends to leave the other party wondering if he/she said something wrong. Ending all calls with warm and polite closures leaves the caller with a good impression of you and your department.

How Did You Rate?

0-10 More than likely, you are contributing to a poor perception of your department and callers are put off by your lack of etiquette. Work on these five areas and your callers will be impressed with the new you. So will your employer.

10-20 Your phone etiquette is mediocre, but you probably slide by without being disciplined. However, you should strive for more than mediocrity and work on creating a more positive impression to all callers.

20-25 Congratulations. When people call and you answer the phone, they're glad it's you. You are polite, accommodating, and provide excellent customer service. You are an excellent model for others to emulate. Keep up the good work.

TOURNIQUET HYGIENE

Have you ever dropped a tourniquet, picked it up, and applied it to your patient's arm?

Have you ever used a tourniquet on a patient that had flecks of dried blood on it?

Is the tourniquet in your tray dull and dingy?

If you were a patient, would you want someone to use your tourniquet—the one on your tray right now—on you?

If you answered "yes" to the first three questions and/or "no" to the last one, it's time to change the way you think about tourniquets. Picking up and using dropped supplies and equipment on your patients destroys their confidence in your willingness to be part of their healing process. It tells them that you are uncouth, unsanitary, and without regard for their well-being. Probably none of these things are true, but that's the message it sends.

Tourniquets can be nasty vectors that carry disease from one patient to another. Don't believe it? Just take your tourniquet to your microbiology department and ask them to culture it. If you reuse tourniquets frequently, what grows will shock you when you see just what you have been planting on the upper arms of your patients.

Nosocomial infections, those spread from patient to patient by hospital staff, are the bane of every healthcare facility. Too often we think that proper hand washing is the only way to combat spreading infection. But discarding tourniquets after several uses is a highly effective way to fight nosocomial infections and help give your patients a fighting chance to avoid a hospital-inflicted infection.

If your tourniquet has flecks of dried blood on it, don't think your patient doesn't notice. And even if he doesn't why would you want to expose him to potentially infectious material? You probably don't, but you might not be used to thinking about it in terms of infection control. If not, take this as a challenge to think about everything you do in terms of infection control, by asking yourself, "What am I exposing my patient to that I wouldn't want to expose my child to?"

Get in the habit of discarding tourniquets that don't look like they've never been used. If they have specks of blood, pitch 'em. If they look dingy, toss 'em out. If you wouldn't put it around the arm of your best friend, don't put it around the arm of a stranger.

Think of tourniquets as disposable; because they are.

OF ALL THE NERVE

Every phlebotomist knows where the veins are in the antecubital area, but do you know where the nerves lie? If you're not sure, don't stick another patient until you are.

Nerve injury is an inherent risk of phlebotomy. Unfortunately, many phlebotomists are never taught the location of the nerves in the antecubital area before they draw patients. As a result, they exercise poor judgment when selecting veins and risky attempts to relocate the needle when they miss the vein. Either of these mistakes can lead to a permanently disabling nerve injury and a lawsuit.

In order to reduce the risk of nerve injury to its lowest degree, all who draw blood specimens must be acutely aware of the location of the nerves in the antecubital area. The most frequently injured nerve is the median nerve, which lies in close proximity to the basilic vein. And if you don't know where the basilic vein is, you shouldn't be drawing blood. Period.

Not all nerve injuries are avoidable, but those that occur because the individual lacks an understanding of the anatomy of the antecubital area not only subject the patient to unnecessary suffering, but the healthcare worker's employer to an indefensible lapse in their training protocol. That means liability. Therefore, whenever collecting blood specimens, keep these tips in mind to fully protect your patient from injury and your employer from a lawsuit:

Because nerves lie adjacent to the basilic vein, probing for this vein should never be attempted.

Because the median nerve can pass over the basilic vein, selecting this vein before ruling out other, less risky veins (such as the median cubital vein) fails to reduce the risk of the procedure to its lowest possible level.

Because a sensation in the patient of a shooting, electrical pain should tell you that you have provoked a nerve, continuing with the venipuncture risks further injury and subjects you and your employer to liability.

Thousands of patients suffer nerve injuries every year during venipuncture procedures.

Most of them are not permanent. But patients whose injury becomes permanent spend the rest of their lives in pain.

Phlebotomy is an invasive procedure; those who insert a needle into the flesh without knowing what lies beneath should not be drawing blood.

BUG BOMBS

Would you take your phlebotomy tray home, set it on your dinner table in several places, remove it, then serve your family dinner on the same table? Of course not! Then why would you place a phlebotomy tray on the same bedside table that a patient eats from?

Think about the surfaces that the bottom of your phlebotomy tray touches during the course of a day: the floor, wastebaskets, countertops where blood is processed and where other trays sit, etc. Imagine the myriad of germs that it picks up in just several hours of regular use and distributes from surface to surface—germs that put patients who are already sick, injured, or unable to fight infection at risk of getting sicker. Multiply that by the number of days since the tray you usually use has been decontaminated. For some this could be weeks; for others, generations.

Placing your phlebotomy tray on a patient's bedside tray is like dropping a bug bomb on their dinner table. Patients use their bedside trays for many purposes besides meals. It's a resting place for dentures, hearing aids, eyeglasses, combs, straws, toothbrushes, arms, and elbows. All of which are capable of delivering to the patient whatever bacteria, fungi, or viruses have been deposited on its surface. Making sure your phlebotomy tray rests elsewhere goes a long way towards minimizing the types and quantities of infectious microorganisms a patient is exposed to.

Instead of using the bedside tray, place your phlebotomy tray on a surface neither the patient nor the patient's personal items are likely to become directly exposed to such as the floor, a chair, etc. Avoid the temptation to place the tray directly on the patient's bed since it may be inadvertently kicked onto the floor by sudden movements. If the bedside tray is too convenient to avoid as a rest for your phlebotomy tray, disinfect the bottom of your tray regularly and/or the patient's tray after use.

Hospitals are places where patients are supposed to get well. We draw blood specimens so that we can contribute to the healing process. Delivering microbes from one patient's dinner table to another's defeats the purpose.

ARE YOU TAKING WORK HOME WITH YOU?

Most people bring home a paycheck from work. If your work involves handling blood specimens, you could be bringing home a whole lot more.

What do you wear when you're processing blood specimens? Are your street clothes protected from splatter or are you taking home the residue of your livelihood to your family? If you draw blood specimens; if you perform bedside testing; remove stoppers from blood specimen tubes; rim clots; transfer blood, plasma, or serum from one tube to another; or otherwise prepare specimens for transportation and/or clinical testing, you should be wearing a protective gown.

In fact, the Occupational Safety and Health Administration (OSHA) demands it. According to the Bloodborne Pathogens Standard, you must wear personal protective equipment such as gowns, gloves, and face shields whenever it is reasonable to expect an exposure. The OSHA Compliance Directive states "laboratory coats or gowns with long sleeves must be used for procedures in which exposure of the forearm to OPIM (blood or other potentially infectious material) is reasonably anticipated." Such coats must be impermeable to blood or OPIM and must be "removed prior to leaving the work area." Translation: wear gowns when working with blood specimens and leave them at work when you go home.

Are you one of those who think that by the time you get home, any blood splatter will have dried and won't be capable of being passed along? If you think that dried blood is dead blood, think again. The virus that causes hepatitis B can survive on environmental surfaces for up to a week.

So next time you drive home after working with open specimens all day without a gown, consider that your clothing could be crawling with critters. So go ahead; hug your kids, embrace your spouse, grab a snack. Just make sure your health insurance is paid up because if you're not wearing a protective gown when you process specimens, you could be taking work home with you.

HAVING A PATHOGEN PITCH IN?

Well, here we go again. It's holiday time. And what do we do more often now than at any other time of the year. We eat. Oh, man, do we eat. In the United States, it's a time of year when we tell the FDA what they can do with their food pyramid and give ourselves permission to declare chocolate as a food group. And when it's time to get ready for that Pitch In at work, the dishes crowd the table like a hundred toy ships huddled together for a bathtub regatta.

If you work in or near a clinical laboratory, you'll agree that labs must have the highest number of refrigerators per capita in the industry. That's a problem the day of the Christmas Pitch In when refrigerator space in the employee lounge is at a premium. But the food keeps coming in and soon someone gets the wild idea that it wouldn't hurt to put their figgy pudding in the chemistry refrigerator just this once, and only until the gorge-fest begins. If you are like-minded, you need to know that OSHA can show up anytime, find your pudding cuddled up between the urine controls and the specimens waiting to be screened for hepatitis B, and in an instant slap your employer with a hefty fine. And that's the good news.

Let's talk about what you are exposing yourself, your co-workers, and your family to when you take the dish home. Did you know that the hepatitis B virus can survive on environmental surfaces for up to a week? So when it's time to set out the culinary delights for the big feast, you could be carrying more to the table than your favorite dish. Think it doesn't happen? Think everyone knows better? Think again. Until 2 years ago, we all thought everyone knew better than to reuse contaminated needles. Then a phlebotomist in California proved us wrong.

According to the Bloodborne Pathogen Standard, "Food and drink shall not be kept in refrigerators, freezers, shelves, cabinets, or on countertops or benchtops where blood or other potentially infectious materials are present."

Can it be any plainer? Undoubtedly, many facilities have an ironclad lock on OSHA compliance and a zero tolerance for employee infractions. For them, it is unthinkable that this reminder is even necessary. In others, lab managers think nothing of storing potato salad with the glycohemoglobin specimens and employee turkeys with frozen serum. Appalling? Yes. Isolated incidents? Don't kid yourself. There are over 10,000 clinical laboratories in the United Sates and hundreds of thousands worldwide. Someone has to occupy the lunatic fringe of the bell curve.

Here's the bottom line: making a holiday exception to storing food in refrigerators that also store biohazardous material—including reagents, chemicals, and blood and blood components—however temporary, is not only uncouth, it's unhealthy and, in the United States, it's a violation of federal standards. Nowhere in OSHA's Bloodborne Pathogen Standard will you find the words ". . .except when there's a Pitch in Dinner."

GLOVELESS PHLEBOTOMY AND THE BLOODBORNE PATHOGENS CLUB

Hey, you! I noticed you're not going to put on gloves for this venipuncture. That's GREAT! Allow me to introduce myself. I'm hepatitis C. I've been watching you and I must tell you how happy I am that you're not wearing gloves. I mean you have no idea how long I've been waiting for someone like you to come along so I can move into your liver and start a family. In fact, you're a perfect candidate for a very elite organization I belong to: the Bloodborne Pathogens (BBP) Club.

The BBP Club needs people just like you. People who think they are so careful when they draw blood that they don't need gloves; people who realize that getting infections from a blood draw is something that happens to other people; people who believe that since they have never gotten exposed to bloodborne infections that they never will be. Is that you? I thought so. You are perfect for us. We need more people just like you to survive. As a member, you're not gonna believe the benefits we offer. Unlimited time off from work; free fatigue; a nice, amber tint to your skin, nailbeds, and the whites of your eyes; HIV cocktails anytime you need them, plus the satisfaction that comes from offering your body to up to 20 different diseases. So, can I sign you up right now? Great! Raise your right gloveless hand and recite the Bloodborne Pathogen Club Creed after me:

- I believe in drawing blood without gloves.
- I believe that my patients don't have any diseases I can catch just by drawing their blood.
- I believe that making me draw blood with gloves is a violation of my civil liberties.
- I believe that yellow, jaundiced skin is quite attractive and that liver transplants are a good thing.

- I believe that my carelessness is my business.
- I believe that those who love me and depend on me don't deserve consideration for how my carelessness will affect them.
- I believe that my skin is perfect and that my fingers and hands never have cuts, abrasions, hangnails, or any microscopic breaks. Never.
- I believe that it's impossible for a needle to come out of my patient's vein accidentally and that I will never have to sop up blood with my bare hands.
- I believe that it's better for me not to report my little accidents than for someone to find out I don't wear gloves.
- I believe that when push comes to shove, I can cut the tip of my glove's finger off and still be able to say I wear gloves.
- I believe I am immortal.

Welcome to the Club!

LABEL OR LIABLE

Pssst. Hey you! Yeah, you. The one who just drew blood from Gladys. You know, that last patient down the hall. I noticed you didn't label the specimens. Let me introduce myself: I'm Gladys' guardian angel. Now, according to my schedule here, she's not ready to be. . .how do you say it. . . "called home" yet. And if you go on as you are, life ends early for Gladys and changes forever for you. I know all this because one of the things that we angels can do is to see the future according to how the present is playing out. And I can see that by the time you get around to labeling Gladys' tubes, you're gonna have someone else's tube in your tray there without a label and you're gonna mix 'em up. I can see it all plain as day.

Don't keep walking down the hall like you don't hear me! I was watching over her when you were drawing her blood. I saw what you did. You put Gladys' tubes in the front left pocket of your scrubs, and her labels in the right one. You know better than that! Look, nobody knows this yet but Gladys has a little mischief going on inside her and she's gonna need blood later on this afternoon. It's all part of the plan, I'm told. We don't ask why, we just make sure everything happens as it should. And what should happen right now is for you to stop stalling and label Gladys' tubes before you take one more step! Because unless I turn things around, that blood you're about to draw from Mr. Jones' is going to end up with my Gladys' name on it and be used for her crossmatch. She'll be dead by morning. Not from her calamity, but from the misfortune of having you leave her room without labeling the tubes. And I just can't have that.

Okay, let's try this: Put your hand in the pocket of your scrubs. Go ahead, put your hand in there. Don't shrug it off. There's something in there. Can't you sense it? Go on, quickly now. Mr. Jones' room is the next one. DO IT NOW!

There you go. Feel the labels? Pull 'em out. There, see? Now go to the other pocket and find the tubes. I was right, wasn't I? Stops you right in your tracks, doesn't it. . .two steps short of Mr. Jones' room. Whew! That was close.

Don't be embarrassed. It happens more than you think. I'm just glad you listened to your impulses. Just remember: Always label specimens at the patient's side. Always!

Don't thank me. I'm your guardian angel, too.

BE SURE BEFORE YOU BANDAGE

Pretend you take an aspirin every day because you've heard it can prevent a heart attack. Or maybe you're on blood thinner. Your doctor has ordered a blood test, so you go to an outpatient drawing center to have a specimen drawn. The phlebotomist draws your blood quickly and without complication and bends your arm up to keep the gauze in place while labeling the tube. The phlebotomist bends your arm back down, removes the gauze, and quickly applies the bandage. You're in and out in less than 3 minutes.

Later that afternoon, your arm aches with increasing intensity. It appears swollen and develops an unnaturally dark color. You check into the emergency room and find that you have been bleeding into your arm from the venipuncture earlier that day. Even though the puncture through your skin sealed, the hole in the vein didn't. They apply pressure and elevate the extremity until they feel confident the bleeding has stopped. You are instructed to stop taking aspirin, limit your activity with the affected arm, and to follow-up with your physician.

Three days later, you see your doctor. Your arm is completely and continuously bruised from your hand to your shoulder. Even though you've followed all discharge instructions, it still aches and you have limited use of the limb. For the first time, your doctor mentions the possibility of amputation.

Think this can't happen? It can and it has. It's not enough to check the puncture site for bleeding on the surface of the skin alone. If you are not checking the site for possible bleeding beneath the surface of the skin, your patient may hemorrhage for hours. Phlebotomists must take time to watch for a raising or mounding of the tissue at the puncture site that suggests the vein is leaking blood into the tissue. It takes less than ten seconds to perform this final visual check before bandaging. Since we don't always know which patients are taking aspirin or blood thinner, it's critical to work this step into our technique.

RESPECT THE NEEDLE

It sends chills down your spine. It changes your life, sometimes forever. It can plunge you into an abysmal depression, thick with uncertainty, doubt, despair, and a gut-wrenching anxiety that consumes every shred of hope for months on end that you'll ever be able to smile without forcing it again.

Not one person who knows will ever look at you the same again. Not your friends, not your family, not your spouse. Although some will come closer to comfort you, some will distance themselves from you in ways that make you feel like a leper who ought not to be touched.

All this because you thought needlesticks were something that happened to other people. You have been drawing blood without an injury for a long time; your technique has been perfected. You are so comfortable with the procedure that you could do it without even thinking about it; then one day you did. Now you can't sleep at night, wondering if there's a virus inside you that you can't stop.

Healthcare workers who respect the needle don't know what this feeling is like. They know the needle is deadly; they won't even recap an unused one with two hands just because they know that if they do, they might allow themselves to do it with a dirty one someday.

Healthcare workers who respect the needle know that every minute of every day, two other healthcare workers get stuck with contaminated needles. At the day's end, over 2,700 other healthcare workers will lose sleep.

Healthcare workers who respect the needle, carry sharps containers to the bedside; they talk as if they are drawing blood absent-mindedly, but their focus is intense and unwavering until the needle is gone for good; they use gloves every time; when drawing with a syringe, they pierce the stoppers without holding the tube with the other hand; they sleep soundly at night.

Respect the needle!

Resources for Managers

A. MINIMUM CONTENT OF ANY SPECIMEN COLLECTION-TRAINING PROGRAM

I.   Critical steps of the venipuncture procedure
    a. Proper patient identification for inpatients and outpatients according to Clinical and Laboratory Standards Institute guidelines
    b. Proper site selection including acceptable and unacceptable sites
    c. Proper antecubital vein selection
      1. High-risk versus low-risk veins
    d. Needle insertion
    e. Tourniquet time
    f. Proper angle of insertion
    g. Order of draw
    h. Tube inversion
    i. Bandaging
      1. Two-point check for complete stasis
    j. Labeling specimens at the bedside
II. Proper capillary puncture procedures
    a. Fingersticks
      1. Acceptable sites
      2. First-drop elimination
      3. Effects of excessive squeezing
      4. Order of draw
    b. Heelsticks
      1. Acceptable sites
      2. Proper prewarming techniques
      3. Squeezing versus forcing
      4. Supplies/equipment removal from crib/blanket
      5. Bandaging restriction

III. Physical risks associated w/venipunctures
    a. Nerve injury
        1. Limits of needle manipulation
        2. Reacting to shooting pain sensation
    b. Hemorrhage
        1. Arterial nick
        2. Incomplete venous stasis
    c. Vertigo/syncope
    d. Lymphedema
        1. mastectomy patients
    e. Over- or undermedication, misdiagnosis, general patient mismanagement

IV. Collection-related analyte alterations
    a. Hemolysis
    b. Dilution with IV fluids
        1. Draws above an active IV
        2. Draws through vascular access devices
    c. Temporary analyte alterations
    d. Posture/diet sensitive analytes
    e. Excessive tourniquet time
    f. Additive carry-over—due to improper order of draw
    g. Pumping fist
    h. Clotting in tubes containing anticoagulants
    i. Contaminated blood cultures

V. Processing-related analyte alterations
    a. Prolonged serum/cell contact
    b. Refrigeration of unseparated clot tubes
    c. Recentrifugation of gel tubes
    d. Delays in transporting/processing sodium citrate tubes
    e. Premature centrifugation
    f. Bilirubin degradation

VI. Practices that increase risk of exposure
    a. Glove use
    b. Removing tip of glove
    c. Dismantling safety features
    d. Failing to use safety transfer device with syringe draws
    e. Forcing blood into collection tubes
    f. Using butterfly needles without a tube holder
    g. No sharps container at the point of use
    h. Overfilling sharps containers
    i. Recapping needles

B. SAMPLE INPATIENT SCRIPT

Statement: "Good morning (afternoon, evening)."
Action: Pause for response.

Statement: "I am (name) from the laboratory. Your doctor would like me to draw a blood sample from you for the laboratory to run some tests. Have you had blood tests drawn before?"

Action: Pause for response. Respond appropriately to patient's reply.

Conditional Response/Action: If the patient requires information about the nature of the test, respond in a general way if you know the nature of the test. Under no circumstances should you provide information about the nature of the test(s) if you are not sure.

Conditional Response/Action: If the patient refuses the test, attempt to explain that the doctor needs the information the test provides to properly treat or diagnose him/her.

Conditional Response/Action: If the patient continues to refuse, do not pursue further. Instead, tell the patient you understand and dismiss yourself. Notify the nurse/caregiver/physician of the refusal.

Conditional Response/Action: If the patient is cooperative, continue by properly identifying the patient.

Statement: "Please state your full name."

Action: Pause for response. Compare information provided with the patient's identification bracelet, which must be attached to their person, and the test form(s).

Conditional Response/Action: If the patient is unresponsive, ask a family member or a caregiver to identify the patient.

Conditional Response/Action: If the arm bracelet is missing or not attached to the patient, notify the nursing staff of the problem. Do not draw the patient until the arm bracelet has been attached to the patient's wrist or ankle or the nurse or caregiver has identified the patient verbally. Document the name of the individual who verbally identified the patient.

Conditional Response/Action: If the patient is unable to state his/her name, seek verification of the individual's identity as above. Document the name of the verifier.

Action: After patient identification has been confirmed, select an appropriate venipuncture site according to facility policy. Prepare the site according to facility procedure and notify the patient of the imminent puncture.

Statement: "You will feel a little poke (alt: 'stick' or 'pinch'), now."

Action: Complete the puncture using the proper order of draw and filling tubes to their stated fill volumes. Release tourniquet, remove the needle, activate the safety feature, and discard the sharp immediately. Apply pressure to the puncture site. Do not allow patient to bend arm up as a substitute for pressure. Invert tubes. Observe for superficial bleeding and hematoma formation. After assuring that bleeding from both the vein and skin has stopped, bandage the patient.

Conditional Response/Action: If the site continues to bleed either above or beneath the surface of the skin, apply 5 minutes of pressure, and then check again for bleeding. If bleeding continues, notify the nurse or caregiver responsible for the patient. Do not bandage the site until bleeding has stopped. Provide patient with post-venipuncture-care card.

Statement: "Here are some instructions for you should you notice anything unusual with the venipuncture site after I leave. I would like to ask you to leave this bandage on for at least 2 hours. Do you have any questions?"

Action: Respond appropriately.

Statement: "Once again, my name is (name). Here's my card with my extension number in case you have any questions after I leave. Thank-you, Mr./Mrs _____."

C. SAMPLE CALLING CARD

```
┌─────────────────────────────────────┐
│                                      │
│        (Your Lab Name)               │
│   ────────────────────────────       │
│        Your Phlebotomist.            │
│                                      │
│     If we can be of further          │
│     assistance, please call. . .     │
│                                      │
└─────────────────────────────────────┘
```

D. SAMPLE POSTVENIPUNCTURE CARE INSTRUCTIONS

General Hospital Laboratory

Thank-you for choosing our laboratory for your blood work. It is our ultimate goal to provide you and your physician with accurate and reliable test results in a timely manner. Your laboratory results will be reported to the ordering physician as soon as they are complete.

Please follow these steps to make sure your venipuncture or skin puncture wound heals quickly and without complications.

1. Leave the bandage on the site for 2 hours.
2. Avoid activities that may put stress on the puncture site, potentially reopening the wound.
3. Make sure you carry your purse or other personal belongings with the opposite hand or arm immediately following the procedure.
4. Avoid lifting and carrying heavy objects for several hours after the procedure.

Rarely, patients can experience complications after a blood specimen is taken. Some potential complications include:

- Bruising at the puncture site

- Bleeding from the puncture site
- Swelling
- Discomfort
- Tingling or numbness in the limb

Should you experience these or any other symptoms you feel are abnormal, immediately contact the specimen collection facility for further instructions.

Should bleeding occur from the puncture site, apply firm pressure and elevate the extremity until the bleeding stops.

Minor bruising is normal and difficult to avoid. However, should you experience abnormal bruising, contact the specimen collection facility for consultation.

Should you feel any discomfort, swelling, tingling or numbness in the limb used in the procedure, contact the specimen collection facility for consultation.

Our phone number is _____.

E. SAMPLE CODE OF CONDUCT

Sample Code of Conduct

(Facility name here) recognizes how important it is to our patients to feel confident that their care has been placed in the hands of caring professionals. We also recognize the value of a professional working environment to our employees. Therefore, (Facility name here) is dedicated to establishing and maintaining this Code of Conduct to which all employees and administrators must comply.

Profanity will not be tolerated. You are not at home. You are in a professional workplace where your speech reflects your integrity and your integrity reflects the quality of work our patients can expect. Use a vocabulary that reflects a more civilized command of the language. Neither patients nor co-workers care to hear offensive language.

Off-color jokes and sexual innuendos are not welcome here. Many of our employees and most of our patients find a haven here from society's preoccupation with sex and crudeness. Please help us keep it that way.

Dress modestly and professionally. Your manner of dress weighs heavily on the image you project. Outlandish colors and styles make patients think that if you can't conform to our dress code, you might not conform to proper procedures either.

Avoid extreme hairstyles, piercing, facial hair, and fingernail treatments. Sure you're an individual, we all are. But don't make patients wonder if you're as cavalier with their bodies as you are with your own. Save the flamboyance for when you're off-duty.

Horseplay is for horses. Don't throw things, ride around in wheelchairs, give each other backrubs, play with equipment, or otherwise goof around. It makes patients think you don't take your work seriously and makes more mature co-workers think they're employed at a daycare.

F. SAMPLE MOTIVATOR ASSESSMENT SHEET

Motivator	RJ	BR	HH	ST	RV	AS	TR	DE	ST	NE	RR	VT	TE	CM
RESPECT														
RECOGNITION														
MONEY														
EDUCATION														
OWNERSHIP														
RESPONSIBILITY														
PROFESSIONAL ENVIRONMENT														
OTHER:														
OTHER:														
OTHER:														

G. TRAFFIC JAM TEAM-BUILDING EXERCISE

Tape a sheet of paper on the floor marked with a large X. (8 1/2" X 11" is fine.) Select 8 volunteers and designate them each as follows: L1, L2, L3, L4, R1, R2, R3, R4. Each participant must remember his or her designation. Line them up as illustrated on either side of the "X". All participants must face in the direction of the "X" in the beginning.

The object is for all participants to move to the opposite side of the "X" using the following legal moves only:

Team members may only move ahead under the following conditions:

1. If the space in front of them is open or;
2. If there is an open space directly behind the person in front of them, one may advance into that open space, but only if the person directly in front of them is facing them.

Players may never move backward.

Allow players to work as a team to achieve the objective.

One possible solution: L1, R1, R2, L1, L2, L3, R1, R2, R3, R4, L1, L2, L3, L4, R1, R2, R3, R4, L2, L3, L4, R3, R4, L4.

Additional Resources **VI**

Relative Centrifugal Force Normogram

To determine the required centrifugal speed for separating serum from cells using gel separator tubes see Figure VI.1 on page 274.

Iontophoresis Equipment

NeedleBuster
Life-Tech, Inc.
4235 Greenbriar Drive
Stafford, TX 77477-3995
Phone: 800-231-9841
Fax: 281-491-6852
Web address: www.life-tech.com

Numby Stuff

Innovative Medical Systems
5950 Shiloh Road East, Suite D
Alpharetta, GA 30005
Phone: 800-972-9705
Fax (770) 886-8110
Web address: www.innovativemedsys.com

RELATIVE CENTRIFUGAL FORCE NOMOGRAM

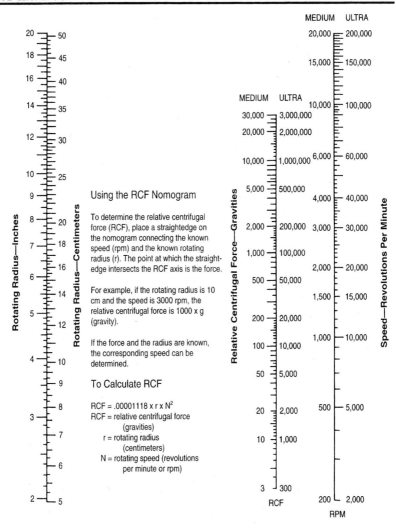

Using the RCF Nomogram

To determine the relative centrifugal force (RCF), place a straightedge on the nomogram connecting the known speed (rpm) and the known rotating radius (r). The point at which the straightedge intersects the RCF axis is the force.

For example, if the rotating radius is 10 cm and the speed is 3000 rpm, the relative centrifugal force is 1000 x g (gravity).

If the force and the radius are known, the corresponding speed can be determined.

To Calculate RCF

RCF = .00001118 x r x N²
RCF = relative centrifugal force
        (gravities)
    r = rotating radius
        (centimeters)
    N = rotating speed (revolutions
        per minute or rpm)

Rotating Tip Radius

The distance measured from the rotor axis to the tip of the liquid inside the tubes at the greatest horizontal distance from the rotor axis is the rotating tip radius.

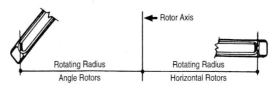

Reprinted by permission from International Equipment Co., Damon Corporation.

FIGURE VI.1

Index

Page numbers followed by "*t*"indicate tables. Page numbers followed by "*b*" indicate boxes. Page numbers in italics indicate figures.